FEEL GOOD, HEAL GOOD

FEEL GOOD, HEAL GOOD

Staying Happy with Homeopathy

DR MUKESH BATRA

BLOOMSBURY

NEW DELHI • LONDON • OXFORD • NEW YORK • SYDNEY

BLOOMSBURY INDIA
Bloomsbury Publishing India Pvt. Ltd
Second Floor, LSC Building No. 4, DDA Complex, Pocket C – 6 & 7,
Vasant Kunj, New Delhi, 110070

First published in India 2024
This edition published 2024

ISBN: PB: 978-93-56406-20-9; eBook: 978-93-56406-22-3
2 4 6 8 10 9 7 5 3 1

Typeset in Adobe Garamond Pro by Manipal Technologies Limited
Printed and bound in India by Thomson Press India Ltd

FSC www.fsc.org MIX Paper | Supporting responsible forestry FSC® C010615

To find out more about our authors and books visit www.bloomsbury.com
and sign up for our newsletters

Contents

For my patients
Because of whom I am who I am and do what I do

Introduction

The significance of mental health has increased tremendously after the Covid-19 pandemic, particularly given the complexities of our modern lives with demanding work environments and performance pressures. Unlike physical ailments, mental health challenges remain hidden—they are not obvious like fevers or coughs and often remain concealed to others behind a facade of normalcy. This concealment is exacerbated by the pervasive social stigma that surrounds mental health issues, making it difficult for individuals to openly discuss their struggles and seek help without fear of judgement.

Mental health significantly influences a person's overall quality of life, affecting not only his or her emotional and psychological well-being but also their physical health. The social implications are profound, as individuals with mental health challenges may face discrimination, isolation and difficulty finding or maintaining employment, which can lead to a further deterioration of their mental state. Relationships, both personal and professional, are also profoundly impacted, as mental instability can strain connections and hinder effective communication. For instance, someone struggling with mental health may find it challenging to secure a job or maintain a positive outlook, which, in turn, can have a domino effect on their overall well-being.

Tragically, the number of suicides, particularly among young people, has been on the rise due to mental illness. Recognising this alarming trend is a crucial step towards addressing the issue of mental health on a broader scale. On 10 October 2023, the World Mental Health Day, it was revealed that 60 to 70 million people in India grappled with both common and severe mental disorders. The gravity of the situation is heightened by the unsettling fact that India holds the unfortunate title of being the world's suicide capital, witnessing over 2.6 lakh cases annually in 2012.[1] These distressing figures underscore the urgent need for comprehensive mental health initiatives and increased awareness to address the escalating mental health challenges in the country.[2]

While there are medications available to manage mental health conditions, such as psychiatric drugs, anti-anxiety medications and sedatives, they often carry the risk of addiction and have a range of side effects. It is important to understand these commonly prescribed mental health drugs and the potential consequences of their long-term use. Selective serotonin reuptake inhibitors (SSRIs) and tricyclic antidepressants (TCAs), for instance, may lead to weight gain. Additionally, these medications can cause sexual dysfunction, digestive issues such as constipation or diarrhoea, and drowsiness that results in fatigue and reduced energy levels. Paradoxically, some drugs prescribed for anxiety or depression may disrupt sleep patterns, leading to insomnia. Nausea, dry mouth, changes in heart rate or blood pressure, tremors and increased anxiety or agitation are among the other potential side effects. These reactions vary among individuals and depend on the specific medication and dosage.

Homeopathy offers a potential avenue for addressing mental health concerns through a holistic lens, acknowledging the connection between the mind and the body. It doesn't isolate symptoms but rather considers them as manifestations of an underlying imbalance. Homeopathic approach and treatments are personalised, aiming not just at alleviating mental distress but also addressing the root cause. Homeopathy values the individual's unique mental, emotional and physical makeup, tailoring remedies to match these specifics. By stimulating the body's innate healing ability, homeopathy seeks to restore harmony, aiming for a long-term well-being rather than just symptom suppression. The approach involves careful listening to understand the patient's experiences, emotions and life circumstances to prescribe remedies that resonate with their overall state, nurturing a holistic path towards providing a remedy for the mental health issues.

Homeopathy provides a safe and holistic system of medicine that can complement traditional treatments. It provides a unique approach to managing various mental health conditions. Promoting awareness of different mental health diseases and available treatment options, including homeopathy, can help reduce the stigma associated with mental health issues and encourage those who are suffering to seek the support and care they need in order to lead healthier and more fulfilling lives.

Clinical Disorders

I

Anxiety

> Anxiety is when the butterflies in your stomach turn into bees.
>
> —Unknown

The word 'anxiety' is derived from the Latin *anxietas*, which means to choke, throttle, trouble or upset. It includes behavioural, emotional and rational responses to the perception of danger. Anxiety is arguably an emotion that predates the evolution of humans. The action of fleeing, which is a part of the flight-or-fight response, is a result of a state of anxiety, and is a primeval trait.

Anxiety is characterised by a host of symptoms, most notably fear, trepidation, inattention, palpitation, respiratory distress, sweating, giddiness and apprehension or fear of death. In certain instances, the root cause of anxiety may be early childhood experiences or situations, especially in school, of being castigated by a stern teacher or bullied by a classmate or senior.

ANXIETY

- In the 1980s the American Psychiatric Association formally acknowledged anxiety as a legitimate mental health condition. Before this, the symptoms of distress due to anxiety were often misunderstood and attributed to general stress or nerve damage. This recognition was a significant step in understanding and addressing anxiety as a psychological issue.[1]
- According to the American Psychological Association, anxiety is a complex emotional state whose features include a sense of heightened tension, presence of worrisome thoughts, feelings of unease, persistent concerns and physical manifestations like elevated blood pressure, accelerated heartbeat and excessive perspiration.[2]

INCIDENCE

- According to the findings of the National Mental Health Survey 2016, approximately 14 per cent of the Indian population needed specific and proactive mental health interventions.[3]
- The World Health Organization (WHO) says that an estimated 38 million people in India are affected by anxiety.[4]
- The WHO states that about 4 per cent of the global population, totalling 301 million people suffer from anxiety disorder. This data ranks anxiety as the most prevalent mental illness worldwide.[5]

FACTS BEHIND IT

- Researchers at the Cleveland Clinic believe that anxiety may result from a mix of different factors including intense or prolonged stress and can affect the chemicals in one's brain that regulate the mood. Being under significant and long-lasting stress for an extended period can eventually lead to the development of an anxiety disorder.[6]

- It is common for an apprehensive person or child to show fear and generalised anxiety or to hold back certain behaviours due to past experience or events. Donning the role of a victim often evokes sympathy and rewards the anxious individual, thus becoming an anti-anxiety defence mechanism for them.
- Anxiety is a normal phenomenon. A certain degree of anxiety or arousal is essential for optimal performance in many situations. At the same time, too little or too much anxiety or arousal leads to suboptimal performance. When a person's anxiety is out of proportion with the requirements of a particular situation, it causes distress and impairs their overall functioning. It is then considered that the individual has an anxiety disorder.

CAUSES

- Hormones
- Excessive stress
- Demands of modern life
- Past traumas
- Heredity
- Medical conditions:
  - Heart disease
  - Diabetes
  - Thyroid disorders
  - Substance abuse

SYMPTOMS

- Excessive worry
- Accelerated heartbeat
- Sweating
- Goose bumps
- Dilation of the pupils
- Paling or flushing of the skin
- Difficulty concentrating

Symptoms of anxiety tend to be persistent and become increasingly worse over time, while flooding their victims with great fear and affecting the quality of their lives with a negative connotation.

Note: Anxiety disorder is quite different from a mild, anticipatory or transitory trepidation that most people experience before a job interview, presentation or important meeting.

TYPES OF ANXIETY

- **Generalised Anxiety Disorder (GAD)**
  Excessive or uncontrollable 'free-floating' worry about a number of events or activities.
- **Panic Disorder (PD)**
  When anxiety is heightened by a sudden thrust, accompanied by palpitation, shortness of breath, increased sweating, trembling, nausea and diarrhoea, with a powerful feeling of imminent doom.
- **Social Phobia or Social Anxiety Disorder (SAD)**
  People believe they are going to be judged negatively or will make a mess of things while speaking in public or meeting new people. It includes excessive anxiety or fear of social situations.

- **Post-Traumatic Stress Disorder (PTSD)**
  Anxiety that occurs after a frightening physical or emotional event, causing the person who witnessed or survived it to have continual, terrifying thoughts and memories or flashbacks of the event.
- **Obsessive–Compulsive Disorder (OCD)**
  OCD, or obsessive–compulsive disorder, is when a person has strong worries or fears that make them perform the same actions over and over again.
  For example, they might repeatedly check if the stove is off, or they may wash their hands many times because they are afraid of germs.
- **Specific Phobia**
  When anxiety presents with excessive or persistent fear of specific objects (e.g., snakes) or situations (e.g., heights or travel by air).

COMPLICATIONS

- **Depression**
  According to WHO, depression is a feeling of persistent sadness and a lack of interest or pleasure in previously rewarding or enjoyable activities.
- **Insomnia**
  According to WebMD, constant worry during the day often carries over into the night. That can cause mental hyperarousal, which can prevent a person from falling asleep.[7]
- **Panic Attacks**
  These are typically present in people suffering from panic disorder (PD). PD is a chronic, frequently disabling disorder. It is characterised by episodic panic attacks that often occur unexpectedly.

Some people with these symptoms avoid all situations that are likely to precipitate a panic attack and so experience few panic attacks. Most people with panic disorder experience coexisting agoraphobia, a fearful anticipation of a variety of situations from which they would find withdrawal or escape difficult. Varying degrees of avoidance may result as a consequence.

People with PD also experience high levels of functional impairment with levels approaching, and in some cases exceeding, those with chronic medical conditions.

PD is generally complicated by other psychiatric conditions, most notably anxiety disorders, depression and alcohol excess. The high likelihood of such coexisting conditions may complicate diagnosis and also treatment outcomes.

Panic attacks may also mimic a wide range of medical conditions. Many of these conditions—cardiac, respiratory, substance- or drug-induced and endocrine-triggered—may have associated signs and symptoms that could alert the doctor to certain underlying factors and assist them in diagnosing PD or differentiating them from others.

In a few patients where such factors may not apply, the doctor may maintain a high index of doubt at initial evaluation. During follow-up, patients who fail to respond as expected to treatment are carefully screened for underlying medical conditions.

Whenever the individual experiences extreme worry, unrelenting fear, social phobia or panic attacks, he or she feels all alone. Nearly 15 per cent of any given population is affected by such overanxious or sometimes panic-ridden feelings.

- **Social Isolation**
  Social isolation is a state of detachment where the person lacks social bonds due to long-standing anxiety.
- **Substance Misuse**
  The National Institute on Drug Abuse estimates that individuals with anxiety are twice as likely to suffer from substance abuse as the general population.[8]
- **Suicide**
  Suicide is a global public health concern. Suicidal thoughts may result due to various mental health issues such as depression, anxiety or substance abuse, as well as social, environmental and personal circumstances like isolation, financial problems and relationship difficulties.

RESEARCH

An epidemiological cohort study from France, reported in *BMC Complementary and Alternative Medicine*, looked at 1,562 patients dealing with anxiety and depression. They were divided into two groups—one group tried homeopathy, while the other group received conventional treatment. The results showed that the patients who used homeopathy needed fewer drugs to felt better and had good clinical progress compared to those who had received conventional care.[9]

HEALING WITH HOMEOPATHY

Anxiety Due To	**Homeopathic Remedy**
Bad news	*Calcarea carbonicum*
Broken love affair	*Ignatia amara*
Business failure/losses	*Ambra grisea*

Anxiety Due To	**Homeopathic Remedy**
Business worries/anticipatory anxiety	*Nux vomica*
Death of near and dear ones	*Natrum muriaticum*
Examination	*Gelsemium sempervirens*
Financial loss	*Rhus toxicodendron*
Good news	*Coffee*
Homesickness	*Phosphoricum acidum*
Domination, in men	*Lycopodium clavatum*
Domination, in women	*Sepia officinalis*
Insult	*Staphysagria*
Jealousy	*Lachesis muta*
Money matters	*Bryonia alba*
Overwork	*Acid picricum*
Post-delivery	*Pulsatilla nigricans*
Stage-fright	*Silicea*
Anxiety Associated With	
Annoyance; irritability	*Nux vomica*
Shock	*Aconite napellus*
Silence	*Natrum muriaticum*
Weeping	*Pulsatilla nigricans*
Fear of death	*Arsenicum album*

Dose: 30C pills, twice a day until symptoms subside.
Please consult your doctor before starting medication.
Specific remedy: *Kalium phosphoricum* 6X, 3–4 tablets, every two hours, till symptoms subside.

CASE STUDY

Sheila, a 38-year-old IT professional, led a contented life with her family. Her work involved long hours in front of a computer, often sitting isolated in her room while striving to meet stringent deadlines. This sedentary lifestyle and extensive screen time eventually manifested in distressing health issues.

Sheila's symptoms began with sleepless nights, coupled with sporadic bouts of anxiety, often accompanied by breathlessness. Her anxiety episodes were triggered by mental exertion and improved notably when she sought solace in open-air surroundings, away from her computer and the confines of closed spaces.

Recognising the need for assistance, Sheila reached out to Dr Batra's, where an extensive case history uncovered the root cause of her anxiety. A pivotal event had occurred eight months earlier when Sheila had a distressing altercation with her mother-in-law, resulting in emotional abuse. This incident left a profound impact, leaving Sheila persistently anxious about her children's future and consumed by an overwhelming fear of death.

In addition to her emotional struggles, Sheila's physical symptoms were meticulously documented. These included a diminished appetite and a heightened thirst for small quantities of water, which provided valuable insight into her overall health condition. After a comprehensive evaluation, encompassing her fear of death, anxiety concerning the future and her unique thirst pattern, the homeopathic remedy *Arsenicum album* was prescribed. Over the course of a month, Sheila exhibited marked improvement, leading to significant changes in her mental and physical symptoms.

SELF-HELP

No one is exempt from some form of mild-to-moderate stress and anxiety at one time or the other. The greater our failure to deal with anxiety and stress, the worse it becomes.

Therefore, how we manage or handle stress and anxiety is important.

The following strategies can help to keep anxiety and stress at bay:

- De-focus on the negatives of the situation.
- Try to bring some enjoyment into your daily activity or take a break from your routine.
- Exercise regularly. Exercise or physical activity is one of the best remedies to reduce anxiety.
  - Scientists at the Anxiety and Depression Association of America found that about five minutes of aerobic exercise can begin to stimulate anti-anxiety effects.[10]
  - Psychologists suggest that a 10-minute walk is as good as a 45-minute workout to relieve anxiety and depression.
  - In one study, researchers found that those who do regular, vigorous exercise were 25 per cent less likely to develop depression or an anxiety disorder over the next five years.

  Vigorous exercise includes:
    - At least 2½ hours of moderate-intensity physical activity (e.g., brisk walking) every day.
    - Each week, 1¼ hours of a vigorous-intensity activity (such as jogging or swimming laps).
    - Jogging, walking, biking, or dancing 3–5 times a week for 30 minutes.

    Setting small, daily, consistent goals helps.
- Interact socially with friends. When you are extremely stressed out, try to remember how you feel when talking to loved ones and/or friends. Get in touch with people you know or don't know, and exchange a smile.
- Pamper yourself with positive feelings, entertain yourself and explore connections with yourself and with

others. Make time for personal interests ('me-time') and hobbies.

- Try to know yourself, the 'real you'.
- Read a humorous book. Or watch a slapstick comedy. Try to laugh and 'laugh your stresses out'. Laughing aloud releases as much endorphins, the feel-good chemical, as a strenuous bout of physical exercise.
- Speak to your professional homeopathic doctor, if or when things go out of control, or you are not able to manage or bring balance to your life with simple lifestyle changes.

Soya, walnut, green, leafy vegetables, potato, milk and milk products, cauliflower, mushroom, cucumber and eggs contain high levels of Tryptophan. These should be consumed in moderation.

2

Depression

> Depression is being colourblind and constantly told how colourful the world is.
>
> —Atticus poetry

ABOUT DEPRESSION

Who discovered depression? In the 19th century, the German psychiatrist Emil Kraepelin started calling different kinds of sadness 'depressive states' because they all shared low mood.

The word 'depression' comes from a Latin word, *depressio*, which means 'to press down or depress'. The term was first used in the literal sense of 'pressing down' in the 1650s. It was also used to describe feelings of sadness and a sinking of one's spirits. It was used as a clinical term in psychology from 1905.

INCIDENCE

According to WHO, depression is widespread as it affects approximately 280 million people worldwide, impacting all age groups. Among children aged 3–17, 1.9 million have been diagnosed. The highest prevalence occurs in individuals aged 18–29 (21 per cent), followed by those aged 45–64 (18.4 per cent), ages 65 and over (18.4 per cent) and ages 30–44 (16.8 per cent).

FACTS BEHIND IT

Depression can physically alter the brain. Research from the United States' National Institutes of Health found that people with depression can lose grey matter volume (GMV) from their brains. This happens because the hormone cortisol can shrink certain parts of the brain and hinder the growth of brain cells. Since GMV holds most of the brain's nerve cells, this could affect the person's thinking abilities.

Every individual's reaction to depression is different. While some may feel sad, others may suffer from symptoms such as restlessness, difficulty in sleeping, unsteadiness, sweating, stomach issues and mood alterations like low spirits, irritability, anxiety or confusion. This is why homeopathy, with its personalised and individualistic approach, is best suited to treat depression. It is also safe, non-addictive and free from side effects.

Depressive symptoms are among the most common complaints in medical practice. Surveys suggest that depression is extremely widespread, with many cases never coming to the attention of doctors.

There is also some conflict between 'normal' depressive symptoms and 'milder' forms of depressive disorders. This is because only the more severe or extreme forms of depression that present with a qualitative distinction from normality get noticed by the family, relatives or friends who are close to the depressed individual.

This is, indeed, one major reason why for homeopathic treatment to succeed, it is always important to know how long the depressed mood has been present, or whether it has been present all the time. Or for how long has it prompted the individual to 'hide themselves away'. Or whether there are thoughts of self-harm or suicidal tendencies. Or whether anything relieves or worsens the depression. Evaluate factors that alleviate or exacerbate depression. Assess if the individual's mood shifts unexpectedly in severity.

Depression may also affect the individual's memory. Although recall of information is unaffected, registration of new material may be challenging.

Depression may affect the person's speed of thinking and movement, too. This is called 'psychomotor retardation'. In severe cases, depressed individuals may not care much about their appearance. This may lead to crumpled clothes or lack of dressing sense.

The depressed individual may often present with a sad and dejected countenance or facial expression. But not always, because in certain cases, the person may put up a brave face and attempt to appear normal. This is called 'smiling depression'. It is therefore imperative for someone in the family or close circle to make an objective judgement based on 'covered outward show' and solicit prompt medical attention for the depressed individual.

A tendency may also be a good pointer in the background of recent life happenings, including the person's cultural and social background and gender. There is a possibility that in some depressed individuals the most perceptible emotion may not be utter despair, but just bad temper or aggression.

Other behaviours that may emerge are poor self-esteem and feelings of worthlessness or guilt. The depressed individual may also impulsively make self-demeaning comments like 'I'm just not good enough'.

It could be beneficial if a family member or someone close gently explores any suicidal thoughts. This may provide reassurance to individuals who might feel overwhelmed by thoughts of ending their own life, possibly leading them to believe they were going crazy or feeling foolish.

If a depressed individual responds favourably to a question such as 'Have things gone wrong so badly that life is not worth living?' one may get some inkling as to whether a 'means' of suicide has been measured. If this is so, one should find out what plans have been made to carry out the attempt or whether they will really act on such intentions. Yet another 'peek' is to figure out whether the person has any hope for the future. The conviction that all is fruitless and that there is no getting away from the present despair, when accompanied by suicidal thoughts, indicates a high risk that such intentions may be acted upon or followed through.

Depressed individuals may experience highs and lows, that is, intense delusions and extremely low moods. These can include beliefs of worthlessness, self-delusions, guilt and excessive worrying about past actions, real or imagined. In severe cases, the depressed individuals may perceive themselves as worse than devils or believe they are responsible for disasters; this is especially prevalent among severely depressed individuals or traumatised soldiers returning from war.

Sometimes, beliefs such as these may lead to persecution of self. In such instances, the depressed person may feel that they deserve to be tormented and punished. In certain cases, the delusory individual may believe that some part of their anatomy has disappeared, withered or 'flushed out' while passing stools.

There may also be hallucinations which may not be as vivid as in schizophrenia, where the individuals can hear certain voices in the ear (*deja entendu*) clearly.

Psychomotor disturbance in the form of slow speech and depressive daze may manifest, along with loss of appetite. There may also be agitation, with repetitive facial appearance of pain and gloom. Physical movements such as wringing of hands, pacing up and down the aisle, along with self-castigation, such as banging the head against a wall or pulling hair (trichotillomania), may be present.

In some instances, there can also be symptoms of anxiety with 'reversed functional shift'. In other words, the individual will not show the usual symptoms of early morning waking, reduced appetite and weight loss. Instead, they may show symptoms of drowsiness, a tendency to sleep all through the day, along with increased appetite and weight gain.

CAUSES

- Childhood traumas
- Stressful life events
- Inappropriate lifestyle such as smoking, drinking, addiction, being into bad company, gambling and always thinking negatively
- Underlying medical conditions
- Heredity
- Financial losses
- Addictions to alcohol, drugs, smoking, internet, video games
- Relationship issues
- Death of loved ones
- Prolonged use of steroids

SYMPTOMS

- Negativity in all aspects of life—a feeling of pessimism, or belief that nothing can make life better
- Changes in sleep patterns—sleeplessness, disturbed sleep, getting up too early or sleeping more than is necessary
- Changes in eating patterns—lack of or change in appetite, or eating too little or too much
- Fatigue
- Difficulty in concentrating or making decisions
- Feeling of isolation
- Withdrawal from people and neglecting one's appearance
- Persistent sadness, self-disgust
- Reduced libido or sex drive
- Failure to experience pleasure (anhedonia)
- Digestive disturbances
- Suicidal behaviour

TYPES OF DEPRESSION

Usually, depression is of two types—exogenous and endogenous.

- **Exogenous Depression**

  This kind of depression is often caused due to circumstances or events and may result from the death of a loved one—a human or a pet. It can also result from job loss or a break in relationship such as separation and divorce. Often, patients in our clinic in London get out of their depression on a pleasant, warm, sunny day. This is called seasonal affected disorder (SAD). Here, people literally go under the weather and become depressed when the skies are grey.

- **Endogenous Depression**
  This kind of depression results from a chemical imbalance in the brain. Neurotransmitters (norepinephrine), which are chemicals released in the brain, trigger this depression.
  Sometimes, the long-term use of chemicals present in Western medicines may also trigger depression, as in the case of anti-hypertensives or blood pressure medicines.
  In women, depression may also be caused by hormones and sometimes can be associated with mood swings before periods (premenstrual tension—PMT) and after delivery (postpartum depression).
  In some cases, depression may also be of unknown origin.

More Than What Meets the Eye

A 46-year-old man from a drug study was referred to a psychiatrist. The patient had both major depression and dysthymic disorder (chronic depression) after a business failure two years earlier. His primary symptoms were increased sleep and decreased enthusiasm, libido, energy and interests. After no improvement during the 'blind' portion of the study, he continued to show little response once the 'code' was broken, and he was treated with two different active, conventional antidepressant medications. He was referred for psychotherapy and further antidepressant trials. The therapy progressed slowly with only episodic improvement. One day, the patient reported that his wife had been teasing him about how, during his afternoon nap, his snoring could be heard over the noise of a vacuum cleaner. The psychiatrist immediately asked additional questions, eventually obtained his polysomnography (sleep study) and, after appropriate treatment for sleep apnea (a sleep disorder characterised by pauses in breathing or periods of shallow breathing during sleep), the patient's depression improved dramatically (Source: Robert Feldman, *Understanding Psychology*, McGraw-Hill).

A Movie about Depression

The film *World's Greatest Dad* tells the story of Lance Clayton, a failed author and high-school poetry teacher. Clayton is seeing a woman who does not want to openly admit their relationship. He also has a drifting, female-obsessed son who loathes him. When his son dies after a gory accident, Clayton arranges his body to make it appear as if he had hanged himself. He then writes a false—but exquisitely poetic—suicide note to avoid embarrassment. The note claims his son killed himself because of depression.

Actually, Clayton is the one who is depressed. His depression helped him write such a beautiful suicide note. Nonetheless, it is his dead son who receives praise and sympathy from peers who read the note and think it is lovely. The community, which once regarded his son as nothing but a jerk and a loser, now applauds him as a gifted poet who suffered from mental illness.

COMPLICATIONS

- **Feeling of Emptiness**
  Feelings of loneliness or sadness or feeling numb or disconnected.
- **Insomnia**
  According to *Johns Hopkins Medicine*, people who have trouble sleeping, like those with insomnia, are at a much higher risk of developing depression—about ten times higher—compared to those who sleep well. And amongst those who are already depressed, 75 per cent of them struggle with falling asleep or staying asleep.[4]
- **Memory Deficit**
  Long-term low moods can lead to memory problems, such as forgetfulness or confusion.
- **Social Isolation**
  The mood swings experienced by depressed individuals make it difficult for them to maintain social connections.
- **Suicide**
  According to research done by the Cincinnati Children's Hospital Medical Centre, over 95 per cent of people who take their own lives have depression or some other diagnosable mental disorder.[5]

RESEARCH

- Depression is one of the most commonly treated conditions by homeopaths worldwide. In a 6-year study of 6,544 patients published in the *Journal of Alternative and Complementary Medicine*, 205 patients were treated with homeopathy for depression. Out of them, 71 per cent showed improvement.[6]

- In another review of 1,783 patient conditions, published in *Homeopathy*, depression was the most frequently treated condition. Among them, 63 per cent of depressed patients experienced significant improvement with homeopathy.[7]
- The *British Homoeopathic Journal* reports that out of 120 psychoneurotic patients treated with homeopathy, 79 per cent improved after six months.
- Dr Jack Cooper, chief psychiatrist in a New York prison, found that homeopathy dramatically improved the health and well-being of treated inmates. Suicides dwindled to zero.
- Homeopathy helps patients who suffer from or have problems related to depression. It has also been shown to reduce related depression in patients having fibromyalgia, or following oestrogen withdrawal in cases of breast cancer.
- Depression accounts for 4–5 per cent of total short-term disability days. In 76 per cent of such cases, the employee is a woman. Reports suggest that employers lose approximately ₹4,500 crore per annum in lost productivity directly related to depression.[8]
- A study published in the *American Journal of Psychiatry* in 2006 stated that an employee with depression averaged 27 lost workdays per year due to absence or poor performance on the job.
- Homeopathy offers a cost-effective, efficacious and safe alternative treatment plan for depression in comparison to conventional medicine, and contributes significantly to reduced lost workdays, without side effects.

HEALING WITH HOMEOPATHY

Depression	**Homeopathic Remedy**
Children	*Calcarea carbonica*
Old people	*Aurum metallicum*
Puberty	*Helleborus niger*
Associated With	
Alone, without others around	*Arsenicum album*
Bad news	*Calcarea phosphoricum*
Cause not known	*Phosphorus*
Coition (after sex)	*Natrum phosphoricum*
Darkness, from	*Phosphorus*
Disappointment in love	*Ignatia amara*
Domestic issues	*Sepia officinalis*
Head injury	*Natrum sulphuricum*
Masturbation	*Phosphoricum acidum*
Music	*Graphites*
Sad stories	*Cicuta virosa*
Smell of flowers, from	*Hyoscyamus niger*
Better/Worse	
Better, weeping	*Phosphorus*
Better, consolation	*Pulsatilla nigricans*
Worse, consolation	*Natrum muriaticum*
Worse, weeping	*Stannum metallicum*

Dose: 30C pills, twice a day until symptoms subside.
Please consult your doctor before starting medication.

Two doses of *Aurum metallicum*, a medicine prepared from metal gold, are useful when self-condemnation and a feeling of worthlessness and despondency are paramount and the patient has a great desire to commit suicide. This medicine is given in its 200 C potency. When such a feeling is causeless, and the patient is irritable and awkward, *Natrum muriaticum*, a medicine prepared from common salt, is very beneficial.

Staphysagria is useful in cases when the feeling results from the ill effects of anger. It is given in its 200 C potency, two doses, once a week.

CASE STUDY

Vijay, a middle-aged businessman, experienced depression due to a large financial loss in his business. He felt burdened by his responsibilities towards his family. He lost confidence, withdrew himself from work and social interactions and lost interest in almost everything in life. His family saw him sinking into severe depression and was worried about his worsening condition. He would avoid going to the office and meeting people. Once a perfectionist, he was now indifferent to his environment. This resulted in a loss of interest in food, family and other day-to-day activities. No amount of encouragement from the family could get him to pull himself together. He consulted many doctors and psychiatrists, but their treatment was only temporarily effective and gave rise to unwanted side effects like drowsiness, dizziness, dryness of the mouth and constipation. A neuropsychiatrist even suggested electric-shock treatment if nothing else worked. The family finally turned to homeopathy. A single dose of *Ignatia amara* helped Vijay overcome his depression within ten weeks. *Ignatia amara* contributed to the resolution of his physical as well as his emotional and gastrointestinal symptoms without any side effects.

In another case, a bright, young man who was a successful management professional would get depressed regularly at work during winter. He would smoke heavily to counter the problem. While analysing his case, it was found that there was a strong sense of rejection, the culprits being his strict, demanding parents and teachers, and this dated back to his childhood. He was given the homeopathic medicine

Medorrhinum. The remedy helped him to overcome his wintry blues and nicotine dependence. It also restored the spark back into his work.

SELF-HELP

- Mayo Clinic advises that exercising at least 30 minutes, 3–5 days a week significantly reduces depressive symptoms as exercising releases endorphins, the feel-good chemicals.[9]
- Progressive Relaxation Exercises
  These exercises help the individual to relax the muscles in their body, one by one.
  Step 1: Start by tightening the muscles in the feet.
  Step 2: Concentrate on slowly letting all the tension go.
  Step 3: Next, tighten and relax the calves.
  Step 4: Continue until the muscles in the body, including those in the eyes and scalp, are relaxed.
- Counselling
  A counsellor can help a person learn to modify or change his or her responses to stress. Psychotherapy can provide significant and long-lasting reduction of symptoms.
- Diet Recommendations
  - Tryptophan is used in treating stress-related depression in patients who have not responded well to other antidepressants. Sources of Tryptophan include dates, milk, yogurt, cottage cheese, meat, fish, poultry, sesame, chickpeas, peanuts and soya.
  - Sugar and caffeine give a quick lift but can leave the person feeling down when their effects wear off.
  - Reducing sugar and caffeine intake helps; feelings of depression often improve when their consumption is minimised.

3
Eating Disorders

> I am beginning to measure myself in strength, not pounds. Sometimes in smiles.
>
> —Laurie Halse Anderson

ABOUT EATING DISORDERS

Eating disorders occur nearly 90 per cent more frequently in women than in men. The cause for this is not known, although eating disorders have no socio-economic, ethnic or cultural associations. Eating disorders affect several million throughout the world, most of them being females between the ages of 12 and 35. There are two main types of eating disorders—anorexia nervosa and bulimia nervosa.

Eating disorders are emotional disorders. A person loses appetite when he or she is under stress. People also tend to substitute emotional deprivation with comfort food—which is why the moment we come home from a long vacation we want to have *dal chawal* (lentils and rice). The mother's cooking is said to be the best, even if it is not good—the feeling of love and warmth with which the food is served is what matters.

- Eating disorders may either lead to weight loss or weight gain.
  - Weight loss: This is not the weight loss which results from diseases (like cancer, tuberculosis, diabetes). This loss results from psychological factors like stress and anxiety, for example, children showing defiance against parents by not eating. They stop eating to tell parents that they are unhappy about something. It is like hitting back. Refusing food is a psychological reaction.
  - Weight gain: In this case, food is a substitute for love and affection. The person eats because he or she is feeling low. Often, parents show love to their children by giving them fast food. When these children grow up, food gets substituted for love for them.
- We celebrate by eating; at the same time, we also try to belong to today's image-conscious society. The result is that obesity and wanting to be thin are major epidemics worldwide.
- All people want to improve their appearance, so starvation diets are common.
- The media drives us to buy certain clothes and products, say, to get rid of our wrinkles and to lose weight. The media gives the message, 'If you lose weight and are thin, you are happy, trendy and loved'.
- The unhealthily thin models in the fashion and film industry are a perfect example of how powerfully our idea of thinness equals happiness. At the same time, the fact is that many of us would benefit from eating a bit less and exercising more to improve our health and fitness levels and keeping illness and disease at bay.

- Watching what we eat is *not* an eating disorder; not watching and eating *is*.
- Eating disorders can be life-threatening illnesses. They can be physical, emotional or psychological in their origin. They result in a range of abnormal and harmful eating behaviours. They are influenced by unhealthy beliefs, perceptions and expectations concerning eating, weight and body shape.
- People with eating disorders have difficulty accepting themselves and feeling good about themselves. They look at themselves as fat and unattractive because of their body size and shape, even though this may not be the case.
- While identifying and defining their perceived obesity, people with eating disorders think they are unacceptable and unwanted. They also have self-doubts and feel inadequate, especially about their bodies. Many of them resort to controlled eating as their best option in their search of thinness.
- If a person has an eating disorder, he or she should know that they are not an exception. Millions of people the world over are overweight or obese. Their number is only expanding
- One important fact is that the individual should not depend on their willpower to get over this condition. Getting a doctor's advice can provide these people with hope of a solution.
- Around 6–20 per cent of individuals with an eating disorder will actually die as a result of their problem.
- Homeopathy looks at the nature of eating disorders, their causes, potential treatments and strategies for prevention. This includes addressing the emotional or psychological underpinnings of the affected individual, along with lifestyle changes and counselling.

- Research indicates that death rates from eating disorders are among the highest for any emotional illness.

ANOREXIA NERVOSA

This presents with self-starvation or a refusal to maintain a minimum normal body weight. Individuals with this eating disorder often engage in self-induced vomiting, use of laxatives, diuretics or excess exercise to control their weight. They also see themselves as overweight, even though they are extremely thin. When the tendency not to eat becomes extreme, death is a lurking possibility.

ABOUT ANOREXIA NERVOSA

The term 'anorexia' was first used in England in 1680 by William Withey Gull, who was Queen Victoria's personal physician. In 1686, Dr Richard Morton described a 20-year-old patient as 'a skeleton covered in skin' in historical medical records.[1]

INCIDENCE

Research indicates that the number of eating disorders in India is on the rise. A 2015 survey by the National Institute of Mental Health and Neurosciences (NIMHANS) revealed that approximately 2 per cent of the Indian population experiences eating disorders. In 2018, another study discovered that around 6.5 per cent of teenage girls in India were affected by eating disorders.[2]

FACTS BEHIND IT

According to the United States' National Eating Disorders Association, several studies have uncovered changes in the serotonin system in people struggling with anorexia nervosa as well as those who have recovered from it. They observed that individuals experiencing anorexia have much lower levels of serotonin byproducts in their cerebrospinal fluid compared to those without an eating disorder.

In a 2009 article in *Nature Neuroscience*, a leading eating disorders researcher, Walter Kaye, suggested that people with anorexia may feel better when they starve themselves because starving reduces serotonin in their brain. However, as they continue to starve, the brain responds by increasing serotonin receptors to use the remaining serotonin more efficiently. This creates a cycle where the person needs to continue to keep starving to feel better. When someone with anorexia starts eating again, serotonin levels suddenly rise, leading to intense anxiety and emotional turmoil, making recovery challenging without proper support.[3]

CAUSES

Some researchers suspect a biological cause for anorexia nervosa and bulimia, such as a chemical imbalance in the hypothalamus or pituitary gland, perhaps brought on by genetic factors. Others believe that the cause has roots in the society's valuation of slenderness and the parallel notion that obesity is undesirable.

Low confidence, depression, anxiety, anger, being alone, troubled family or personal relationships, emotional problems, being taunted about size or weight and physical abuse are some other causes of eating disorders.

Other factors may include cultural pressures that celebrate size-zero and thinness as the perfect body, not to speak of biochemical or biological variants, besides a family history of eating disorders.

SYMPTOMS

- General
  Body image disturbance
  Dietary habits—food restrictions
  Eating behaviour—eating slowly, eating in isolation
  Others like excessive exercise, induced vomiting as well as misuse of laxatives, medications and drugs
- Physical
  Dizziness, syncope
  Fatigue
  Abdominal pain, constipation and bloating
  Absence of menstrual cycles in females
- Psychiatric
  Self-harm
  Suicide
  Anxiety and depression
  OCD

COMPLICATIONS

Cardiological	Bradycardia Hypotension	– Slower heart rate – Low blood pressure, which causes fainting or dizziness because the brain doesn't receive enough blood
Psychiatric	OCD Anxiety Depression	– Excessive thoughts (obsessions) that lead to repetitive behaviours (compulsions) – Feelings of sadness, hopelessness and reduced energy, nervousness, worry

Structural	Low BMI Muscle wasting Hypothermia	– BMI under 18.5 is considered to be low, i.e., underweight – Loss of muscle mass due to the muscles weakening and shrinking – A significant drop in body temperature occurs in people suffering from eating disorders due to a reduction of fat tissues

RESEARCH

Research suggests people with anorexia nervosa and bulimia become used to their weight and feel bad that they can't lose more and be thinner. Some psychologists suggest that eating disorders result from overly demanding parents or other family problems. The complete explanations for anorexia nervosa and bulimia, however, remain elusive.

HEALING WITH HOMEOPATHY

Anorexia	**Homeopathic Remedy**
Fear of becoming fat	*Natrum muriaticum*
Fear of being poisoned	*Hyoscyamus niger*
Hormonal disturbances	*Sepia officinalis*
When people fast to pacify God	*Veratrum album*
With Craving For	
Alcohol, tobacco	*Medorrhinum*
Chocolates	*Argentum nitricum*

Dose: 30C pills, twice a day until symptoms subside.
Please consult your doctor before starting medication.

CASE STUDY

Anil, a 16-year-old boy with a history of anorexia and previous hospitalisation, embarked on a journey of higher education in a different city after successfully completing his 12th board exams. During his two-year stay in a hostel, a troubling pattern emerged. He would bring his hostel meals to his room but instead of consuming them, he stashed the food in various corners of his room. For one and a half years, he restricted his diet to water, tea and juices, resulting in a substantial weight loss of 20 kg. Alongside his drastic diet, Anil developed peculiar actions such as constant hand and foot washing, a reluctance to leave the hostel and interact with people and a strong belief that he was being ridiculed at college, which ultimately led to avoiding classes. He also engaged in obsessive behaviours, frequently weighing himself and exercising excessively whenever he imagined he had gained weight. Anil was prescribed *Natrum muriaticum* based on his fear of gaining weight, a preference for solitude and his clear symptoms of obsession. The primary change observed after starting *Natrum muriaticum* treatment was a gradual restoration of his appetite. Anil began to eat his meals regularly and his mental state progressively improved. He took the initiative to dispose of the weighing machine himself. Following these positive developments, Anil received counselling in addition to homeopathic treatment. This comprehensive approach contributed to his remarkable recovery, and he regained 12 kg during the treatment.

SELF-HELP

- Don't diet haphazardly; design a meal plan that gives all the nutrition the body needs.

- Take advice from a professionally qualified dietician.
- If your loved ones say you are normal weight, thin or fat, believe them.
- Prioritise self-care such as getting enough sleep, engaging in relaxation techniques and participating in enjoyable activities.

BULIMIA NERVOSA

Individuals with this disorder possess uncontrollable eating pattern, often accompanied by inappropriate methods of purging to remove food from their system before it can be fully processed.

ABOUT BULIMIA NERVOSA

The term 'bulimia' has its roots in late Middle English, evolving from *bolisme* to *bulimy*, and is ultimately derived from the Greek word *boulimia*, which means 'ravenous hunger'. It combines *bous* (ox) and *limos* (hunger).

INCIDENCE

NIMHANS says that eating disorders impact an estimated 2–3 per cent of the Indian population, with a higher occurrence among women.[4]

FACTS BEHIND IT

The University of California San Diego Eating Disorders Center's researchers suspect that abnormal serotonin levels may heighten susceptibility to bulimia.[5]

CAUSES

- Genetic Factors
  The Eating Disorders Centre says that bulimia is believed to arise from a genetic predisposition influenced by life events and family environment.[6]
- Biological Factors
  Studies have shown a higher prevalence of bulimia in individuals with a background of obesity or a family history of eating disorders among parents, siblings or other close relatives.[7]
- Emotional Factors
  People who experience depression, anxiety, loss of a loved one, separation, incidents of sexual or physical abuse or bullying can develop bulimia.[8]

SYMPTOMS

- Self-induced vomiting
- A tendency to 'binge and purge' privately (individuals having bulimia often maintain normal or above the normal body weight—this is because they try to conceal their purging bouts from others, including family and friends)
- Recurrent episodes of binge eating
- Fear of not being able to stop eating
- Inappropriate use of laxatives or diuretics
- Inflamed and sore throat due to constant vomiting
- Erosion of teeth enamel from vomiting

COMPLICATIONS

Medical

- Weight fluctuations
- Nutritional deficiencies
- Gastrointestinal damage (from laxative abuse)

- Electrolyte abnormalities (from laxative and diuretic abuse as well as vomiting)
- Fluid loss resulting in dehydration

Social
- Poor body image, particularly when paired with strict dieting
- Suicidal thoughts and attempts
- Low self-esteem
- Depression

RESEARCH

In a 9-week pilot study published in *Alternative Therapies in Health and Medicine*, researchers at the University of Johannesburg investigated the use of individualised homeopathic remedies to address binge eating in 15 male participants. The study assessed changes in binge eating intensity and frequency using a binge eating scale. The findings of this study stated that individualised homeopathic treatment reduced both the intensity and frequency of binge eating in the sample studied.[9]

HEALING WITH HOMEOPATHY

Bulimia MED	**Homeopathic Remedy**
Precipitating Factors	
Grief or major disappointment	*Ignatia amara*
Guilt	*Staphysagria*
Trepidation, often related to weight	*Carcinosin*
With Craving For	
Alcohol, tobacco	*Medorrhinum*
Chocolates	*Argentum nitricum*

Dose: 30C pills, twice a day until symptoms subside.

Please consult your doctor before starting medication.

CASE STUDY

An overweight medical student, Rani, sought help for recurrent depressive episodes that had been going on for four years. Her primary concern was her unhealthy eating habits. These issues began during her early days in medical college when she developed affection for a classmate who, unfortunately, rejected her. This rejection had a profound impact on Rani, leading to a deep dissatisfaction with her body and appearance. She began to perceive herself as overweight, which prompted her to skip meals and only consume salads. Over time, she lost 12 kg. To reduce her weight, she resorted to taking isabgol husk, a laxative, to purge after overeating. To fund a liposuction procedure, she even sold her gold necklace without informing her family.

Upon obtaining her medical history, Rani was prescribed *Ignatia amara* considering her disappointment. Although she initially hesitated to take the prescribed doses, even sporadic use of the medication began to help her address her inner conflicts and she gradually improved her eating habits. Alongside homeopathic treatment, Rani received counselling to develop self-acceptance. With consistent follow-up sessions, she found relief and eventually overcame her emotional turmoil.

SELF-HELP

- Always believe that being healthy overall is better rather than focusing on weight.
- Plan balanced meals with the help of nutritionist.
- Avoid skipping meals as that can contribute to cravings and increase the risk of overeating.
- Leptin, an appetite suppressant, is a hormone produced by fat cells that signals satiety.

Some foods naturally stimulate leptin and boost your metabolism, for example, grapefruit, whole grains, soya, legumes, broccoli, egg yolk, nuts and carrots.

WEIGHT LOSS

INCIDENCE

According to WHO, approximately 1.9 billion adults are overweight, while 462 million are dealing with underweight issues.

On a global scale, in the year 2020, approximately 149 million children under the age of 5 experienced stunting (being too short for their age), 45 million faced wasting (being too thin for their height) and 38.9 million contended with overweight or obesity.[10]

CAUSES

Mental Conditions

- Depression
- Anxiety
- OCD
- Eating disorders

Problems with Digestion

- Coeliac disease
- Irritable bowel syndrome (IBS)
- Poor absorption of nutrients
- Increased metabolic rate

Other Health Conditions

- Prolonged illness
- Overactive thyroid

- Diabetes
- Heart failure
- Tuberculosis
- Cancer
- Peptic ulcer
- Substance abuse (alcohol, cocaine, others)
- Prolonged use of medications
  - Hydralazine: high blood pressure medications
  - Antibiotics such as penicillin
  - Methylphenidate: ADHD
  - Digoxin: Heart medications
  - Chemotherapy medicines
  - Antiepileptic drugs such as topiramate, felbamate and zonisamide

SYMPTOMS

- Loss of appetite
- Infections
- Abdominal bloating or abdominal pain
- Chronic constipation
- Difficulty swallowing
- Loose or painful teeth
- Mouth soreness

COMPLICATIONS

- Dehydration
- Slow metabolism
- Muscle wasting
- Nutrient deficiencies
- Death

HEALING WITH HOMEOPATHY

Weight Loss	**Homeopathic Remedy (to gain weight)**
Extreme weakness, lassitude, reduction in strength of body leading to weight loss	*Oleum jecoris*
Localised weight On thighs and buttocks On abdomen	*Lycopodium clavatum* *Natrum muriaticum* *Calcarea carbonicum*
By burning fat tissues	*Fucus vesiculosus*
By increasing metabolic rate	*Phytolacca*
To regulate thyroid gland functioning	*Thyroidinum*

Dose: 30C pills, twice a day until symptoms subside.
Please consult your doctor before starting medication.

CASE STUDY

Mayuri, a 35-year-old woman, experienced a significant and concerning postpartum weight loss of 8 kg. Rather than embracing the joy that typically accompanies the arrival of a new life, she found herself grappling with depression as a result of her drastic weight loss. In an effort to regain the weight she had lost, Mayuri embarked on various diet plans and weight gain programmes, but she saw no progress. Recognising the need for a more in-depth evaluation, she underwent a thyroid function test, which indicated hyperthyroidism. She was prescribed a homeopathic remedy *Thyroidinum*. Remarkably, within just one month of commencing this treatment, not only did Mayuri gain 10 kg, but her depression symptoms were also significantly alleviated.

SELF-HELP

- Set a motivational goal.
- Resist strong cravings, make healthy choices.
- Be mindful of the portion size.
- Eat more fruits and vegetables.
- Avoid higher-calorie foods that provide less nutrition.
- When you have hunger pangs, distract yourself for five to ten minutes.
- Replace food with fresh fruit and avoid junk food.
- Stay hydrated.
- Avoid drinks with added sugar.
- Alcohol adds up calories.
- Do light exercises lift some weight.
- Get enough sleep.

WEIGHT GAIN

ABOUT WEIGHT GAIN

- The term 'diet' is derived from the Greek word *diaita* which emphasises a healthy lifestyle focused on both mental and physical well-being, rather than being confined to a narrow weight-loss regimen.
- The first widely recognised dietary plan was the 'Banting' diet, named after William Banting.

  In his 1863 pamphlet titled 'Letter on Corpulence, Addressed to the Public', Banting introduced a detailed low-carbohydrate, low-calorie diet that had helped him reduce his weight significantly.[11]

INCIDENCE

- India is grappling with an obesity epidemic, facing one of the world's most rapidly increasing rates. Current estimates suggest that approximately 135 million individuals in the country are affected by obesity.[12]

- According to the World Heart Federation, current global estimates indicate that approximately 2.3 billion children and adults are dealing with obesity. Alarmingly, if the current trends persist, it is projected that the number could surge to 2.7 billion adults grappling with overweight or obesity by the year 2025.[13]
- The World Obesity Atlas for 2022, released by the World Obesity Federation, projects that 1 billion people worldwide will be contending with obesity by 2030, that is, 1 in 5 women and 1 in 7 men globally will be living with obesity.[14]

FACTS BEHIND IT

Every 10 kg of extra weight reduces life by three years according to the International Federation for the Surgery of Obesity and Metabolic Disorders.[15]

According to the WHO, excess of body fat significantly increases the risk of non-communicable diseases, including 13 different types of cancer, type-2 diabetes, cardiovascular issues and respiratory conditions. Alarmingly, in 2021, obesity contributed to a staggering 2.8 million deaths on a global scale.[16]

Obesity as a psychological condition was not part of the early or old psychiatric classification. Today, it is—even when most cases of obesity do not fulfil the necessary criteria for inclusion as a psychiatric disorder or as a clinically significant behavioural or psychological syndrome that causes distress or disability.

While overweight is defined as 'abnormally high body weight due to excessive accumulation of body fat', there are certain ethnic differences in the distribution of subcutaneous fat. But the general cause of the disorder is plain overeating. Besides this, excess weight may also result from abnormal retention of water, unusual muscular development and some tumours, as well as a few endocrinal disorders.

Global Epidemic

Excess weight is a global epidemic. It is a disease, a sign of illness—a complex syndrome. Thanks to its growing incidence, obesity is being studied as closely as any other disease.

Research mentions genetic, emotional, metabolic, sociological and environmental factors as causative factors. Excess weight also has a strong predisposition in children. Some endocrinologists suggest that the hereditary aspect may not be largely congenital, that is, present at birth, although final overweight, or excess weight, may be a direct consequence of 'the clean plate syndrome' which some mothers persevere with as a rule for their children.

Overweight problems arise primarily in relation to your attitude to food, weight and body size. They also project your emotional status—whether or not you have a rigid approach to eating and/or exercise. Your eating habits can make or break your health and happiness. The longer the belt, as it is rightly said, the shorter the life.

Fat people are often thought of as jolly, good folks. They are also identified as candidates for an early heart attack. The hazards of being overweight are serious.

Role of Diet

Research states that if you substantially reduce the intake of calories, without reducing your nutritional intake, you will live longer. In addition, you will remain healthier with fewer health issues or illnesses. Fads diets don't help. Also, don't go by the big promise of miracle diets, or magic pills.

If you are serious about reducing your weight, you need to speak to a professional homeopathic doctor—never self-treat yourself. The purpose is not losing weight alone, but keeping it down, and also remain healthy in the long-run.

Exercise

While you are reducing your intake of food, without compromising on your nutritional intake, it is critical that you also increase your physical activity in consultation with a trainer or coach. This will not only decrease your waistline, it will also help your heart and lungs to work better, improve your mood, give you a sound night's sleep and decrease your risk of serious illness or disease. Relaxation techniques, such as yoga and meditation, are just as useful—they help to ease your level of stress, which is also one of the primary causes of obesity.

CAUSES

- Lack of physical activity
- Unhealthy eating habits
- Consuming food high in fat and sugar
- Disturbed sleeping pattern
- High amounts of stress
- Heredity
- Prolonged use of steroids
- Medical conditions:
  - PCOD
  - Depression
  - Hypothyroidism
  - Heart problems

SYMPTOMS

- Reduced power and stamina
- Lethargy
- Excess belly fat
- High blood pressure
- Weight gain
- High cholesterol
- Joint pains

Types of excess weight:
- Overweight: BMI 25 to 30
- Obesity: BMI 30.0 or higher

COMPLICATIONS

Life expectancy of overweight individuals, after the age of 35, is often associated with a death rate much higher than that of people with normal weight.

Increased body weight causes:
- High blood pressure, high cholesterol, diabetes mellitus, stroke
- Low quality of life
- Depression, anxiety and other mental disorders
- Body pain and difficulty with physical functioning

RESEARCH

International clinical trials have shown that certain homeopathic remedies act as fat burners; they stimulate and accelerate the body's metabolic process, without side effects.

According to a study published in the *Tantia University Journal of Homoeopathy and Medical Science*, homeopathic medicines address underlying medical, hormonal and psychological factors contributing to obesity, along with the complications caused by obesity. Homeopathic medicines play a role in weight management by enhancing digestion, metabolism and the elimination of waste.[17]

HEALING WITH HOMEOPATHY

Weight Gain	**Homeopathic Remedy**
A pot-bellied child or adult with craving of eggs and thyroid problems	*Calcarea carbonicum*
Thyroid enlargement in obese people	*Fucus vesiculosus*
Obesity with anaemia, puffy face and pitting of flesh	*Ferrum metallicum*
Fat and sluggish persons with large bodies and large buttocks	*Ammonium muriaticum*
Obese females with paleness and thyroid, uterine fibroids or mammary tumours	*Thyroidinum*
Tendency to grow fat easily with longing for acids and pickles	*Antimonium crudum*
Obesity in females with delayed menstruation	*Graphites*
A moody, overweight lady who loves junk food	*Phosphorus*
Aversion to fatty foods, still grows obese	*Pulsatilla nigricans*
Ravenous hunger after heartbreak	*Natrum muriaticum*
Weight gain from sedentary lifestyle	*Nux vomica*

Dose: 30C pills, twice a day until symptoms subside.
Please consult your doctor before starting medication.
Specific remedy: *Phytolacca mother tincture*, 8–10 drops in half a cup of water, twice a day, half an hour before meals (for losing weight).
Alfalfa Q, 20 drops in half a cup of water half an hour before meals to improve appetite.
Oleum jecoris 6C, 5 pills twice a day half an hour before or after meals.

CASE STUDY

Jason, a 50-year-old male, came forward with concerns about his excess weight and fluctuating thyroid and cholesterol levels. He had been taking conventional medications for years to manage these problems. The unique pattern of his symptoms appeared to be associated with mental stress, as his symptoms tended to worsen when under stress. In response to his specific symptoms, Jason was prescribed *Fucus vesiculosus*. After a few months of treatment, he experienced significant improvements in his weight management, his long-standing thyroid problems and his cholesterol levels, all of which eventually reached acceptable levels.

SELF-HELP

- Set an inspiring goal.
- Pay attention to eating habits.
- Be doubly sure about the portion size and choice of food.
- Avoid high calorie food.
- Develop a strategy to control weekend binging or excesses.
- Avoid sedentary habits.
- Eat a healthy mix of proteins and carbohydrates; consume oats, wheat, jowar and ragi.
- Avoid meats and meat products containing high amounts of fats; prefer fish or lean meat instead.
- Avoid sweets and sugary foods as they spike sugar levels.

4

Attention Deficit Hyperactivity Disorder (ADHD)

ADHD is like having a racecar brain with bicycle brakes.

—Unknown

ABOUT ADHD

Emotional and psychological illnesses are increasing in number especially anxiety, depression, attention deficit hyperactivity disorder (ADHD) and autism. These illnesses are the result of the pressures of modern-day life.

INCIDENCE

According to a study published in the *Open Journal of Psychiatry and Allied Sciences*, research conducted in Assam indicated a prevalence of ADHD ranging from 2 per cent to as high as 17 per cent.[1]

In terms of numbers, an article published in *India Today* stated that approximately 10 million Indian children are diagnosed with ADHD each year.[2]

CAUSES

- Behavioural specialists suggest that there may be a connection between the amount of time children spend watching TV, learning disabilities and ADHD. We can also add time spent on mobile phones, computers and video games. This also results in short-attention spans that many of our children exhibit.
- Research suggests that the rapid shift of visual frames on TV is related to the hyperactivity syndrome. This occurs because of non-stop camera flips and varied spotlights, where the viewer's thought-compass changes every few seconds. With short-attention spans the hyperactive child is attempting to recall the dynamic quality of the TV screen by quickly changing their own perceptual points of reference.
- A slight diminishing of mental capabilities is almost universal after a certain age. Usually minimal, it can be ignored in most cases. In some people however, this failure may be extreme or at an earlier age. This might affect the individual's career prospects. Lack of concentration, very common amongst school and college-going children, in individuals with pole-vaulting ambitions and in those involved with figures, affects writing and reading comprehension. This can be a serious impediment to the person's functioning. Worry, tension and anxiety are common causes for lack of concentration.

SYMPTOMS

- The primary symptoms include inattention, hyperactivity and impulsivity.
- Impulsivity is characterised by:
  - Short reaction time

  - Low inhibition
  - Failure to learn from previous experiences. This may precipitate risk-taking behaviours with impairment to the child's well-being. This may also warrant constant supervision of the child.
- For ADHD to be confirmed, symptoms should have begun before the age of seven and should have been present for at least six months. Hyperactivity consists of motor restlessness, fidgety temperament, overactivity on the move and restlessness, independent of a social context. The symptoms may continue even during sleep.
- ADHD symptoms include:
  - Difficulty following instructions
  - Inability to maintain focus—in academic work or play activities in school and at home
  - Tendency to misplace or lose things needed for activities at school and home
  - Appearing inattentive
  - Not giving close attention to detail
  - Being disorganised; trouble planning ahead and executing tasks
  - Forgetting things quite easily; getting easily distracted; losing track of thoughts

COMPLICATIONS

- Trouble interacting with and being accepted by peers and adults
- Increased risk of alcohol and drug abuse
- Pattern of negative behaviour towards authority figures
- Antisocial behaviour such as stealing, fighting, destroying property and harming people or animals
- Frustration

- Overwhelming worry and nervousness
- Manic behaviour

RESEARCH

The *European Journal of Pediatrics* published a three-phase study on ADHD. In the first phase, children were prescribed a homeopathic constitutional remedy. Those who improved by at least 50 per cent on the ADHD rating scale proceeded to the second phase, which included a placebo group. Subsequently, the children resumed their homeopathic remedies, and their progress was monitored for four weeks. In the third phase, the children were randomly assigned to receive either the appropriate homeopathic remedy or a placebo.

The study's results revealed that children did not experience improvement with the placebo but continued to show progress with the homeopathic remedy.[3]

HEALING WITH HOMEOPATHY

ADHD	Homeopathic Remedy
Restless child, likes to move around continuously	*Tuberculinum*
Restless child, likes dancing to loud music	*Tarentula hispanica*
Restless, aggressive or violent individuals	*Mercurius solubilis*
Restless, with extreme fear	*Stramonium*
Moves hands with restless intensity	*Kalium bromatum*
Moves feet constantly; restlessness of limbs mostly	*Zincum metallicum*
Restless, but feels safe in the most dangerous place	*Agaricus muscarius*
Dull or slow child	*Calcarea phosphoricum*

ADHD	Homeopathic Remedy
Nervous and impulsive person	*Argentum nitricum*
Recent onset accompanied by fear	*Aconite napellus*
Restlessness resulting from grief and mental shock	*Phosphoricum acidum*
Tendency to get lost in thought, marked loss of concentration	*Sulphur*

Dose: 30C pills, twice a day until symptoms subside.
Please consult your doctor before starting medication.

CASE STUDY

Mathew, a 9-year-old boy, had been struggling to maintain concentration even for short periods. He found it challenging to concentrate on his studies without getting distracted every 10–15 minutes. Mathew's teachers frequently commented on his poor concentration. Interestingly, Mathew's lack of concentration wasn't evident when he was playing or watching TV, but mainly surfaced during exams or study hours. He tended to immerse himself in his own thoughts. Despite trying various nerve-tonics as recommended by their family physician, there was no improvement. Mathew was prescribed a single dose of *Sulphur* to address his lack of concentration and his habit of getting lost in his own thoughts. His parents were also advised to spend more time with him. After two months, his parents reported significant progress. Mathew could now study for longer periods and maintain focus for extended durations.

SELF-HELP

Parents can take several actions to help their child:

- Set clear goals, give specific commands.

- Don't give confusing instructions.
- Praise the child's accomplishments.
- Parent–child relationship is the most important part in the development of the child.
- Do not curse or blame the child. Help him to overcome the situation.
- Encourage outdoor activities.
- Limit screen time.
- Try games that challenge the brain.
- Always shower a lot of love and affection on the child.

FREQUENTLY ASKED QUESTIONS: ADHD AND HOMEOPATHY

Homeopathy considers each child as being different from another child. What causes a problem in one may not cause it in another. Homeopathy assesses each child and treats him or her based on their unique characteristic temperament and exhibited or latent symptoms.

New research suggests that most behavioural disorders in children are metabolic in nature; they are not essentially emotional disorders.

To succeed one must, therefore, first aim to correct the child's metabolism. Homeopathy aims to improve the child's behaviour and learning ability by giving a suitable homeopathic remedy that boosts bowel function. This, in turn, improves metabolic and brain function.

Q: How can homeopathic remedies help children with intellectual and developmental disabilities?

A: Intellectual and developmental disabilities often include a variety of conditions like emotional problems, ADHD, dyslexia, autism and Down's syndrome. Such kids tend to suffer from a host of physical and psychological problems with high incidence of epilepsy, obesity, poor dental health, side effects of conventional drugs, and so on. With their inability to cope with their peer group and society, the likelihood of traumatic events, such as abandonment by loved ones, abuse, bullying and mental harassment, is also often high. This may leave a deep negative impact on them. Homeopathy, due to its stimulating, therapeutic action on the mind and body, helps to resolve such problems naturally. Most important, homeopathic remedies are simple, easy-to-take or administer and free from side effects.

Homeopathic remedies, such as *Kalium bromatum* and *Tarentula hispanica* are not only clinically useful to ease ADHD-triggered restlessness and temper tantrums, they also improve attention span, and thus improve academic performance.

Studies published in the *British Homeopathic Journal* and the *European Journal of Pediatrics* report that ADHD children who were given homeopathic treatment showed significantly less ADHD behaviour.

Q: How early should parents take their hyperactive children for homeopathic treatment?

A: Any deviation in behaviour in comparison to 'normal' kids of the same age or siblings should alert parents to consult a professional homeopathic doctor. This is because there is generally a significant time lag between the appearance of symptoms and establishment of the diagnosis. It is, therefore, always better to start the treatment early.

Q: Can homeopathic remedies help in speech and behavioural problems too?

A: Children with speech and behavioural problems tend to be angry or depressed and/or experience mood swings due to their inability to cope with peer pressure and surroundings. In addition, symptoms such as restlessness, lack of concentration, temper tantrums and impulsiveness are also common.

Professional homeopathic treatment helps such kids to cope better, calm down, improve their self-esteem and attention span and reduce impulsivity and restlessness. Speech therapy, or supportive learning therapy, may also be given in conjunction with homeopathic remedies like *Baryta carbonicum* or *Calcarea carbonicum*, as the case may be. The two are clinically effective in behavioural problems of children.

Q: What can be done to create awareness and popularise homeopathic treatment for ADHD and other behavioural disorders?

A: Training teachers and parents to identify behavioural problems right in the early stages and encouraging them to seeking medical help is imperative. In addition, making parents and others aware that professional homeopathic treatment is safe and effective for ADHD and other behavioural problems is important. This will encourage parents to opt for early treatment for their child.

5

Obsessions

> Good requires motivation, great requires obsession.

ABOUT OCD

Obsessions are persistent and recurrent urges or thoughts that lead to anxiety and distress. Obsessions result in obsessive-compulsive disorder (OCD). OCD is an anxiety disorder characterised by two core symptoms—obsessions and compulsions. Obsessions are thoughts, images or ideas that won't go away, are unwanted and cause extreme distress. Compulsions are behaviours that a person feels he or she must carry out over and over again.

OCD is socially, emotionally and vocationally more than unnerving. It can at times be very dangerous. There are individuals who are excessively 'clean'. They are perfectionists and can't stop tidying up a place or washing their hands frequently.

OCD is one of the most common of psychological disorders. Its representation extends from being underplayed to being glamorised. It is, in fact, diagnosed as often as asthma and diabetes. Out of every ten individuals visiting a psychiatrist's office, one is likely to be suffering from OCD.

INCIDENCE

The National Mental Health Survey 2015–16 reported that 150 million Indians suffer from mental illness including depression, anxiety and OCD out of which 1 per cent of the population showed concern over suicidal risk.[1]

CAUSES

- Research suggests that a person's genes may play a role in the development of the disorder, although no specific gene for OCD has been identified yet. Studies have identified four brain genes for OCD.
- OCD tends to run in families. When a parent has OCD, there is an increased possibility that their child may develop OCD, although the risk may be low.
- The genes play a role in the same brain circuit. This may help explain why people are more likely to have OCD if they have a relative with the condition.
- OCD has both psychological and neurobiological components. For example, having insufficient levels of serotonin—a neurochemical found in the brain—could be a likely neurobiological factor.
- Among the psychological factors, a primary underlying cause according to Sigmund Freud's theory is the suppression of mental trauma in the past or during childhood. Sometimes, rigid upbringing may also trigger OCD.

SYMPTOMS

- The obsessive personality is characterised by over-conscientiousness, tidiness and a tendency to pay a great deal of attention to detail.

- Obsessions and compulsions are often associated with a marked degree of shame. This may lead many of those afflicted by OCD to hide their symptoms and suffer in silence.
- Those affected can't stop wiping their hands absolutely clean at every step, checking their door locks or praying again and again.
- Performing such rituals, however, provides temporary relief.
- Likewise, not going through such rituals may tend to markedly increase the anxiety.

COMPLICATIONS

- OCD may lead to clinical depression over a period of time.
- OCD may increase the intensity of bouts of low spirits, frustration or a sense of hopelessness.
- OCD may interfere with day-to-day life, producing difficulties at work, finances and also relationships.

RESEARCH

A study highlights the role of homeopathy in the treatment of OCD. According to research published in the *Indian Journal of Research in Homeopathy*, personalized homeopathic treatments have demonstrated effectiveness in treating OCD.[2]

HEALING WITH HOMEOPATHY

OCD	Homeopathic Remedy
Checks, rechecks the house door and lock	*Arsenicum album*
Continuously checks and rechecks things	*Tuberculinum*

OCD	Homeopathic Remedy
Irresistible tendency to be suspicious and jealous	*Lachesis muta*
Washes face constantly	*Pulsatilla nigricans*
Washes hands constantly	*Medorrhinum*
Thoughts of having committed a crime and is about to be arrested	*Zincum metallicum*
Always feels guilty of crime	*Aurum metallicum*
Loves bathing	*Calcarea sulphurica*
With sexual thoughts	*Platina (Platinum metallicum)*
Thoughts of suicide	*Aurum metallicum*
Guilt from depression	*Psorinum*
Continuous depressing thoughts	*Natrum muriaticum*
Ruminations of God	*Cannabis indica*
In women the situation aggravates at the time of periods	*Sepia officinalis*
Over-obsessed perfectionist	*Carcinosin*

Dose: 30C pills, twice a day until symptoms subside.
Please consult your doctor before starting medication.

CASE STUDY

Arvind Billimoria, a man in his mid-40s, suffered from recurrent colds. He would get a sore throat and a running nose. The attacks were very frequent and left him quite weak. On further inquiry, it was found that he was very fond of sweet things and warm drinks. Temperamentally, he was sensitive and emotional. He was a very loving person. He was doing well in his job as the chief executive of his firm. He was also a very meticulous person. He disliked dirt and untidiness and could not rest without cleaning and putting things in their right place. This was a matter of concern because all the time he would clean things around him twice over to make sure there was not even a speck of dust on them. He would point out constantly to his family members if things were not arranged and placed the way he had decided. This fastidiousness became a source of irritation in the family. Two doses of *Arsenicum album* of 200 C potency were given to him every week for a month.

After a month Billimoria reported that the bouts of cold had reduced. He also found himself more relaxed. He was then prescribed two doses of the same medicine per month for two months. In his next visit, Billimoria happily informed that his meticulousness had reduced to an extent which did not upset him or his family members.

SELF-HELP

- Understand that obsession cannot be reduced at once—it takes some time.
- Try to slowly reduce the amount of time spent on carrying out the OCD activity.
- Try to wash hands quickly; don't keep on doing so for several minutes.
- Quickly check the lock, switches, and so on, rather than checking them repeatedly.
- Make a checklist which can satisfy OCD symptoms.
- Cut down screen time.
- Get adequate sleep as poor sleep can trigger OCD.

6

Fears

> Thinking will not overcome fear, but your actions will.

Fear, medically referred to as a phobia, is an instinctive, frightened reaction to a situation or stimulus which is out of proportion to the danger presented by that particular situation. An individual may be prone to such fear because of several factors. Occasionally, physical distress such as sweating, coldness of the body, internal trembling, a sinking sensation or diarrhoea may accompany such an attack. Generally, patients tend to rearrange situations so that they are able to avoid the fear-inducing stimuli. Such avoidance, however, may upset growth and development, thus disturbing one's peace of mind. Medical and psychological help in such a situation is a must.

ABOUT FEARS

Phobias, fears and anxieties have a long history. The first recorded phobia dates to around 600 BC.

The Byzantine Emperor Heraclius had an irrational fear of large bodies of water, particularly those in which he could potentially drown.[1]

INCIDENCE

According to the *Indian Journal of Psychiatry*, nearly 50 million Indians face phobic disorders.[2]

FACTS BEHIND IT

According to *Neurology Live*, people with phobias show increased amygdala activity when exposed to fear-triggering stimuli, as seen in functional MRI scans. A study found that higher right amygdala activity corresponds to greater distress from phobia triggers.[3]

CAUSES

- Negative experiences
- Genetic link
- Changes in brain functioning

SYMPTOMS

- Dizziness, shaking of the body, palpitations
- Difficulty thinking about anything other than the fear
- A powerful impulse to get out of the situation
- Persistent worrying about upcoming events that involve the phobic object or situation

COMPLICATIONS

- Social isolation
- Avoiding places and things of fear
- Mood disorders
- Substance abuse
- Suicide

RESEARCH

According to a study published in the *International Journal of High Dilution Research*, a series of five case reports of patients treated by homeopathy for phobia in the outpatient department (OPD) of the National Homoeopathy Research Institute in Mental Health, Kottayam, were analysed using the American Psychiatric Association (APA) Severity Measures for Phobia Adult over the course of a year. The average severity measure value for these five cases, which was 35 at the beginning, reduced to 0 (indicating asymptomatic) within an average duration of 8 months. Improvement continued steadily up to 12 months with the application of individualised homeopathic treatment.[4]

HEALING WITH HOMEOPATHY

Fears	Homeopathic Remedy
Fear of Dark (Nyctophobia)	
Accompanied with fear of approaching death	*Cannabis indica*
With hallucinations that he or she is surrounded by black insects	*Stramonium*
Fear of Dogs (Cynophobia)	
Fear of dogs	*Belladonna*
Fear of Crowds (Agoraphobia)	
Fear of death, of going out	*Aconite napellus*
Fear of crowds	*Thuja occidentalis*
Fear of Hospitals (Nosocomephobia)	
Fear of going to hospital because he or she thinks they are in last stage of disease	*Arsenicum album*
Fear of Pregnancy or Childbirth (Tocophobia)	
Fear of death from pain	*Coffea cruda*

Fears	**Homeopathic Remedy**
Fear of Dreams (Oneirophobia)	
Fear of sleeping and frightful dreams	*Nux vomica*
Fear of Suffering (Pantophobia)	
From some terrible internal disease	*Lilium tigrinum*
Patient feels cough is intolerable and that death is preferable	*Syphilinum*
From stroke, heart disease or high blood pressure	*Kalium arsenicum*
Fears of heart disease; fears he or she is incurable	*Lilium tigrinum*
Of approaching death, that he or she will die of suffocation	*Spongia tosta*
Fear of Cancer	*Agaricus muscarius*
Fear of Heights (Acrophobia)	
Fear of height and of flying in airplanes	*Argentum nitricum*
Fear of Closed Places (Claustrophobia)	
When going through a tunnel or similar closed space	*Stramonium*
Fear of Open Places (Agoraphobia)	
Fear of open places, nervous about public appearance	*Gelsemium sempervirens*
Fear of Water (Hydrophobia)	
Accompanied with convulsions on thinking of water; where a person wants to drink water but is unable to do so	*Lyssinum*
Fear of eating or drinking, with delirium	*Hyoscyamus niger*
Fear of Failure (Atychiphobia)	
Fear of failure with weak memory	*Lycopodium clavatum*
Fear with Hopelessness	*Aurum metallicum*
Fear of Sex	
In women	*Kreosotum*

Fears	Homeopathic Remedy
In men, with suppressed sexual desire, history of rape or sexual abuse	*Staphysagria*
Other Fears	
Reluctant to appear in public	*Gelsemium sempervirens*
Trains	*Succinum*
Poverty	*Bryonia*
Injury	*Stramonium*
Own shadow	*Staphysagria*
Knives, forks and all pointed things	*Spigelia*
Women	*Pulsatilla nigricans*
Being poisoned	*Hyoscyamus niger*
Dentist	*Gelsemium sempervirens*
Rain	*Elaps corallinus*
Fire	*Cuprum metallicum*
Thunderstorms, darkness or animals	*Argentum nitricum*
Fear of trivialities accompanied by anxiety	*Aconite napellus*
Fears develop without any noticeable cause	*Valerianum officinalis*
Exam blues	*Aethusa cynapium*

Dose: 30C pills, twice a day until symptoms subside.
Please consult your doctor before starting medication.

CASE STUDY

Rajan, a 30-year-old man, had been dealing with claustrophobia. Once he had got trapped in his office elevator for some time. This caused him to develop an unnatural fear of confined spaces. As a result, he began avoiding projects that involved travel or crowded places. In terms of his temperament, he was timid, sensitive, touchy and moody. A physical examination revealed the presence of warts on his neck, and he was both short and overweight. Considering these observations, Rajan was prescribed a single dose of *Thuja occidentalis*. In his subsequent visits, Rajan showed significant improvement. He even travelled alone by train without experiencing fear. After completing the course of treatment, Rajan reported no further episodes of claustrophobia, signifying a successful outcome with homeopathic intervention.

SELF-HELP

- Try not to give in to fear and run away from the situation.
- Talk openly—open communication with loved ones and confronting the issue head-on can facilitate resolution and understanding in the face of challenging events or problems.
- Open up about your phobia—it can help.
- If talking openly is uncomfortable, try writing things down.
- Remember, panic attacks are exhausting; try coping with them.
- Relaxation techniques such as meditation, breathing and stretching can help immensely.
- During attacks, focus on breathing to come out of the situation.

Non-clinical Disorders

7

Anger

> You will not be punished for your anger; you will be punished by your anger.
>
> —Buddha

ABOUT ANGER

Interestingly, the word 'anger' can be traced to the Old Norse word *angra*, which means to feel sad or upset. This word likely comes from an even older word in a Proto-Germanic language, where 'angus' meant something painful.[1]

One of the early thinkers who studied anger and how to handle it was the Roman philosopher Seneca (around 4 BC to AD 65). Seneca observed and learned about anger and ways to control. This was an early version of anger management.[2]

INCIDENCE

A study titled 'Aggression among Adolescents' published in the *Adesh University Journal of Medical Sciences & Research* found that 51.9 per cent of young people showed signs of being aggressive, where boys tended to show physical aggression more and girls showed more hostility.[3]

In a Gallup poll, 160,000 people were surveyed in 116 countries during 2020 and early 2021 to understand the world's mood. This global emotional report revealed that in 2020 more people felt stressed, sad, angry and worried than in the past 15 years, making the world a sadder and more stressful place.[4]

A study by the Harvard Medical School and Teaching Hospital found that about 22 million Americans have a quick-temper problems.[5]

FACTS BEHIND IT

Being angry and stressed can shorten one's lifespan. A research study by the University of Michigan conducted over 17 years discovered that couples who keep their anger bottled inside tend to have a shorter life than those who openly express their anger.[6]

CAUSES

Anger often stems from irritability, which manifests when frustrated. In children, it may lead to temper tantrums, signalling emotional maladjustment if frequent or intense, indicating an inability to tolerate delayed demands. The roots of irritability are often found in one's family background, with tense family atmosphere and anxious, high-strung parents contributing to it. Additionally, abnormal relationships and certain parental attitudes can lead to irritability in later life. In some cases, changes in brain electrical activity, influenced by factors like hypoglycemia, over-breathing or dehydration, may contribute to irritable behaviour in unstable individuals.

Some other causes of anger are:

- Stress
- Feeling of insult, disrespect
- Lack of acknowledgement or unfair treatment
- Financial challenges
- Work or relationship issues
- Violence or abuse

SYMPTOMS

Symptoms include repeated, sudden episodes of impulsive, aggressive, violent behaviour; angry verbal outbursts; grossly disproportionate reactions to situations; and involvement in aggressive acts that are out of proportion to the triggering circumstances.

TYPES OF ANGER

- Behavioural anger
- Chronic anger
- Passive anger
- Judgemental anger
- Verbal anger
- Volatile anger
- Self-abusive anger

COMPLICATIONS

- **Anxiety**
  Anxiety is a feeling of nervousness, unease and worry. Suppressed or unexpressed anger can be an underlying cause of anxiety and depression.

- **Depression**
  A study outlined by *JAMA Psychiatry* considered over 500 people with major depression and discovered that over half of them displayed noticeable anger and irritability, which was linked to more severe and long-lasting depression.[7]
- **High Blood Pressure**
  Chronic anger can lead to elevated blood pressure levels which is known as a sign of the body's fight-or-flight response.
- **Insomnia**
  A study from Iowa State University shows that if you sleep only a little less at night than required, you're likely to be angrier and have trouble dealing with frustrating situations compared to those who get enough rest.[8]

RESEARCH

According to the *International Journal of Health Sciences*, constitutional homeopathic treatment is effective in management of anger. Homeopathy reduces violence and makes the life of the patients healthier and happier.[9]

HEALING WITH HOMEOPATHY

Anger Due To	Homeopathic Remedy
Disappointment in love	*Natrum muriaticum*
From contradiction	*Sepia officinalis*
In head-strong and haughty people	*Lycopodium clavatum*
In bad-tempered people	*Matricaria chamomilla*

Dose: 30C pills, twice a day until symptoms subside.
Please consult your doctor before starting medication.

CASE STUDY

Ayush, a 6-year-old boy, was the only child of his parents. He was the centre of their attention, especially because he was born after 10 years of his parents' marriage. As he grew up, he became very demanding and irritable, especially when he was touched. This behaviour caused chaos at home and in public. Ayush's parents decided to try homeopathy to help him with his irritability and touch sensitivity. After a single dose of *Chamomilla*, there was a significant improvement. He became less demanding and irritable and his aversion to being touched decreased. He became more cooperative and started sharing his feelings more openly with his family. This success with homeopathy strengthened his parents' trust in the treatment.

SELF-HELP

- Take deep breaths when anger is uncontrollable.
- Deep breathing can normalise racing heartbeats and high blood pressure.
- Count from 100 to 1 in reverse order.
- Pause and think before you speak.
- Avoid engaging in arguments; try keeping mum.
- The *Aggressive Violent Behavior Journal* states that changes in the brain's dopamine levels can make people more impulsive and prone to aggression. Dopamine helps a person to stay calm and not lose temper. If someone has low dopamine, they might get angry or become aggressive easily. To boost dopamine, in your daily diet you can incorporate fruits and vegetables like apples, bananas, oranges, watermelon, strawberries, avocados, beets, tomatoes, green leafy vegetables, as well as milk and dairy products.[10]

8

Emotional Disorders in Children, Teens and Seniors

> You don't have to control your thoughts; you just have to stop letting them control you.
>
> —Dan Millman

EMOTIONAL DISORDERS IN CHILDREN

BREATH HOLDING

This can be frightening and alarming for the parents as the child becomes lifeless and unresponsive.

INCIDENCE

According to *Indian Pediatrics*, up to 27 per cent of growing children may exhibit breath holding spells.[1]

According to research, approximately 5 per cent of the population experiences breath holding spells between the ages of 6 and 18 months.[2]

CAUSES

- Iron deficiency, anaemia
- Fatigued or overtired child
- Change in the child's breathing
- Slow heart rate

SYMPTOMS

During episode, the child gives out one or two long cries and then holds his or her breath until the lips and face become bluish with stiffness of the body.

- Fainting, usually within less than a minute
- Temper tantrums
- Getting scared
- Sudden injury, such as by falling down
- Muscle twitching or a seizure
- The symptoms only appear when the child is awake, never when asleep.

COMPLICATIONS

- Serious complications of breath holding spells are rare
- Sudden death
- Absence of heartbeat (asystole)
- Seizures

HEALING WITH HOMEOPATHY

Breath Holding Spells	**Homeopathic Remedy**
Associated With	
Behavioural disorders	*Ignatia amara*
Dentition	*Matricaria chamomilla*
Night terrors	*Stramonium*

Breath Holding Spells	Homeopathic Remedy
Respiratory problems	*Mephitis putorius*
Anaemia	*Ferrum phosphoricum*

Dose: 30C pills, twice a day until symptoms subside.
Please consult your doctor before starting medication.

CASE STUDY

A 3-year-old boy was brought to the clinic for an evaluation of breath holding spells. The first episode occurred six months before the clinic visit when he had a minor accident at the poolside, hitting the back of his head. During this incident, he did not lose consciousness and recovered by himself, although he appeared pale. Subsequently, the child started experiencing episodes where he would lose consciousness and turn blue. This would often happen before school. Aside from these spells, he was generally healthy, with a history of anaemia. Initial assessments, including a CT scan and EEG after the first episode, gave normal results. A complete blood count was conducted to rule out iron deficiency, which revealed low haemoglobin levels. During a detailed discussion with the parents it was discovered that the child intentionally triggered these episodes to avoid going to his kindergarten school. A treatment plan involving *Ignatia amara* was given to address his hysterical behaviour and counselling was recommended, which led to positive outcomes in a relatively short time.

SELF-HELP

- Check the child's mouth for food or any object that could cause choking during the spell.
- Placing a cold, wet cloth or splashing cold water on the child's face can shorten the episode.

- Episodes can occur if children are upset or hurt.
- Stay calm during the episode.
- Don't force your child to breathe during the episode. Breath holding spells usually end within a minute.
- Take prompt action if something unusual is sensed.
- Try to avoid child becoming too hungry or overtired.
- Adequate sleep is recommended.

FITS OF ANGER

INCIDENCE

A Harvard study revealed that approximately 1 in 12 teenagers may be affected by an anger disorder. Almost 8 per cent of them exhibit recurrent, severe violent outbursts.[3]

CAUSES

- Childhood dominating episodes
- Traumas

SYMPTOMS

- Rage
- Irritability
- Continuous/uncontrollable agitated thoughts
- Tingling
- Tremors
- Palpitations
- Chest tightness

COMPLICATIONS

- Impaired interpersonal relationships
- Frequent verbal and physical fights

- Self-harm
- Medical complications:
  - Blood pressure
  - Diabetes
  - Heart disease

HEALING WITH HOMEOPATHY

Fits of Anger	**Homeopathic Remedy**
Jealousy from sibling rivalry	*Hyoscyamus niger*
Extreme rage leading to biting	*Stramonium*
Raving and ranting	*Hepar sulphur*
Desire to tear and cut things with scissors	*Veratrum album*
Obstinacy and restlessness if demands are not met	*Matricaria chamomilla*
Associated With	
Contradiction	*Aurum metallicum*
Destruction	*Tarentula hispanica*
History of mental and physical abuse	*Staphysagria*
Restlessness and hyperactivity	*Tuberculinum*

Dose: 30C pills twice a day until symptoms subside.
Please consult your doctor before starting medication.

CASE STUDY

A 5-year-old boy, Ashu, was brought by his mother to the clinic regarding his skin issues and anger problems. Ashu had a tendency to get angry quickly, particularly when things did not go his way. His anger manifested as loud complaints, arguments and even hitting. He also had feelings of jealousy towards his elder sister. On a physical level, he exhibited teeth grinding, scaly skin eruptions, a strong desire for sweets and strong dislike for some foods. In his dreams, he seemed to be engaged in some sort of a battle, frequently telling someone to leave him alone. After a detailed assessment of the case, Ashu was prescribed *Tuberculinum* based on a strong dislike for a particular food item, dreams, anger, jealousy, and so on. Following a single dose, Ashu's argumentative behaviour decreased significantly, and he became less aggressive. His sleep quality improved and he was no longer troubled by his dreams. Overall, he became a more relaxed and contented child, excelling in both his school and social life. Furthermore, he developed a strong creative side in his extracurricular activities, demonstrating confidence and composure while achieving success in various aspects of his life.

SELF-HELP

- Self-help for fits of anger involves managing intense, impulsive outbursts, while self-help for general anger focuses on coping with displeasure and resentment in a more controlled manner.
- According to psychologists there is a simple FIVE-S method for kicking out unhealthy anger:
  - **Stop**
    Stop thinking about yourself, how you feel, what you've done.
  - **Shift**
    Shift your focus to the present moment. Ask yourself, 'What can I do right now to make things better?'
  - **Set a Goal**
    What outcome do you wish to achieve?
  - **Strategise**
    What are some ways to achieve that goal?
  - **Start**
    Begin action towards achieving your goal.

ATTACHMENT DISORDERS

> Attachment is root of all sufferings.
>
> —Popular saying

ABOUT ATTACHMENT DISORDERS

Attachment theory was first introduced by John Bowlby, a British psychologist and psychiatrist. This is a psychological, evolutionary and ethological theory that provides a descriptive and explanatory framework for understanding interpersonal relationships between human beings. There were some preliminary papers from 1958 onwards but the full theory was published in the trilogy *Attachment and Loss*, 1969–82.[4]

Attachment is a dynamic process. It is biologically driven and is mutually reinforcing and adaptive for the parent and the child. The progression boosts loving care and growth of emotional warmth and bonding of the parent and the child. It also enhances positive associate relationships between parent and the child.

INCIDENCE

According to Cleveland Clinic, 1–2 per cent of children suffer from attachment disorder where they do not form an emotional bond with their caregivers. This includes adopted children.[5]

FACTS BEHIND IT

Research published in *Frontiers in Behavioral Neuroscience* indicates that maternal care can affect the hypothalamic–pituitary axis, potentially impacting behaviours. Similarly, disruptions in parent–child relationships in the child's first two years can have a significant influence on a child's psychological development and behaviour.[6]

Mother–Baby Attachment Theory: In Freud's psychoanalytic theory, attachment development was linked to the gratification by the mother of a child's instinctual drives. According to Freud, the emotional connection between the mother and child emerges because the infant attaches to the mother as the source of nourishment.[7]

CAUSES

- Attachment need not necessarily be biological, that is, to mother or father. It can occur with outsiders too, including babysitters if they take part in the interpersonal processes that enable adjustment and closeness-seeking experiences.
- Attachment behaviour is also a relational process. It arises as a result of the behaviours of both the infant and the parent, or caregiver. This is the central principle because, theoretically, attachment disorders may result due to a shortfall or malfunction in relations, which may be because of the caregiver or the child, or both.
- A key clinical feature of attachment disorders is the inability of the child to distinguish and focus on key caregivers in later childhood. For the caregiver too, an insufficient response to infant signals and inability to provide an encouraging environment—physical and/or emotional—is the central aspect.
- Sometimes a child's needs are met and sometimes they aren't. The child never knows what to expect leading to disbalanced behaviour.

- An infant or young child is hospitalized or separated from the parents.
- Death of both or either one of the parents.
- The parent is emotionally unavailable because of depression, illness or substance abuse.
- Abusive, strict parent.
- Abuse, maltreatment and trauma experienced by the parent or the child.
- Differently abled parents.

SYMPTOMS

- Unexplained withdrawal, fear, sadness or irritability
- No response when comfort is given
- Aversion to touch and physical affection
- Affection is perceived as a threat

COMPLICATIONS

- Reluctance to obey rules or cooperate
- Non-compliance with collaboration or teamwork
- Feelings of anger and bitterness
- Slower development
- Delayed or slower language acquisition
- Repetitive behaviours
- Behavioural issues
- Struggle in academics

HEALING WITH HOMEOPATHY

Attachment Disorder	**Homeopathic Remedy**
Due to family discord or childhood traumas	*Magnesium carbonicum*
As a result of shock or a negative experience	*Aconite napellus*
Due to fear of being alone	*Calcarea carbonicum*

Attachment Disorder	Homeopathic Remedy
Due to separation	*Pulsatilla nigricans*
Due to suppressed emotions, past unfortunate events	*Staphysagria*

CASE STUDY

Ritu, a precious little girl born to her parents after 15 years of marriage, faced a unique challenge. Her father worked abroad, and the family resided in India. Due to his work commitments, her father could only take one-month leave each year to be with Ritu. During this time, she would cling to him, but as his vacation drew to a close, she experienced increasing discomfort. Initially, she felt sadness when he had to depart, but this evolved into episodes of breathlessness. After a thorough evaluation, it became evident that these episodes were closely linked to her father's departure, highlighting a strong sense of separation anxiety. She was prescribed *Magnesium carbonicum* to address the separation dilemma. Additionally, her father was advised to extend his stays for the sake of her well-being. Over time, the severity and frequency of these episodes reduced and eventually she bid her departing father a happy farewell, demonstrating the positive impact of addressing her separation anxiety.

SELF-HELP

- Shower love on the child.
- Rocking, cuddling, holding hands and simple gestures make a big impact.
- Respect the child's needs.
- Take your child to a garden, sanctuary, zoo and so on.
- Help the child to play outdoors and relax.

- Avoid screen time on mobile phones and computers.
- Pamper the child in every possible way.
- Acknowledge and appreciate the child for his or her good work.
- Ensure healthy diet for optimal brain health.
- Make the sleep schedule (bedtime and waking up time) consistent.
- Take psychological counselling as and when needed.

BEDWETTING

ABOUT BEDWETTING

Bedwetting has been referred by ancient Egyptians in 1550 BC. In papyrus writings from that time, as a remedy, they mentioned using sugar cane, known for its liquid-absorbing properties. The fibres of sugar cane were used to make a potion to combat bedwetting. The effectiveness of this lay in the sugar cane fibres' capacity to absorb excess water from the bloodstream. This signalled the kidneys to store fluid due to a perceived deficiency to maintain the body's fluid balance. Consequently, the rate of urine production slowed down, facilitating nighttime restraint because the bladder received a lower volume of fluid.

Interestingly, the drug *Minirin*, used to treat bedwetting since the early 1980s, operates on a principle similar to the one discovered by the ancient Egyptians more than 3,500 years ago, underlining the enduring wisdom of this ancient approach.[8]

INCIDENCE

According to the *Indian Journal of Nephrology*, a comparative study was done at a few centres where 1.4–28 per cent of children aged 6–12 years suffer from enuresis globally. In

India nocturnal enuresis has been reported in 18.4 per cent of children from a single centre.[9]

FACTS BEHIND IT

According to a research study published by WebMD, it has been observed that reduced levels of anti-diuretic hormone (ADH) in children is responsible for bedwetting. ADH is responsible for instructing the kidneys to produce less urine. The diminished quantity of hormone released during sleep is associated with an increased volume of urine, which contributes to the occurrence of bedwetting.[10]

CAUSES

- Nocturnal enuresis is evidenced to be hereditary. It tends to run in families. Nearly 70 per cent of parents who were late in becoming dry may have a child with incontinence. Twins are twice as likely to be affected.
- A small bladder
- Inability to recognise a full bladder
- Deep sleeper
- Hormonal imbalance
- Recurrent urinary tract infections (UTIs)
- Interrupted breathing, especially during sleep
- Chronic constipation
- Developmental defects

SYMPTOMS

- Involuntary urination
- Nightmares
- Sleepwalking with a full bladder

COMPLICATIONS

- Guilt and embarrassment
- Social isolation
- Cannot take part in any camps or overnight stays due to fear of bedwetting
- Infection or fever due to sleeping in wet undergarments
- Urinary retention

RESEARCH

An observational trial study conducted in the outpatient department of the Calcutta Homoeopathic Medical College and Hospital was reported in the *Indian Journal of Research in Homoeopathy*. This study focused on individuals aged 5 to 18 years experiencing nocturnal enuresis. A total of 34 participants were enrolled, and their scores were recorded on bimonthly basis. The most commonly prescribed medicine during the trial was *Kreosotum*. The results showed that homeopathic medicines offer a promising treatment option for individuals with nocturnal enuresis.[11]

HEALING WITH HOMEOPATHY

Bedwetting	**Homeopathic Remedy**
Adolescents	*Lac caninum*
Boys	*Rhus toxicodendron*
Old men	*Aurum metallicum*
Weak children	*China officinalis*
Women	*Silicea*
Precipitating Factors	
Anxiety	*Kalium phosphoricum*
Catheterisation	*Magnesium phosphoricum*

Bedwetting	Homeopathic Remedy
Fright	*Aconite napellus*
Habitual	*Equisetum hyemale*
Head injury	*Silicea*
Nervousness	*Gelsemium sempervirens*
Worms	*Cina maritima*
Time of Recurrence	
First sleep	*Sepia officinalis*
Towards morning	*Ammonium carbonicum*
Winter	*Causticum*

Dose: 30C pills twice a day, until symptoms subside.
Please consult your doctor before starting medication.
Specific remedy: *Verbascum* Q (Mullein oil) 20 drops, in half a cup of water, one hour before bedtime

CASE STUDY

Parth, a 7-year-old child, was brought to the clinic by his parents for his persistent bedwetting. His mother diligently woke him up once or twice during the night, but the bedwetting problem persisted. The parents tried various home remedies and tricks but nothing worked. During a detailed case analysis, it was discovered that Parth had a deep fear of his strict father, which was likely the trigger for his bedwetting. Additionally, he would frequently wake up in the middle of the night in a state of fright, possibly due to frightening dreams. Based on this analysis, he was prescribed *Aconite napellus* to address his anxiety and fear of his father. After four months of treatment, Parth's bedwetting became a thing of the past and he experienced significant improvement in his frightening dreams and fear of his father.

SELF-HELP

- Try inculcating dry bed training by:
  - Reducing the amount of fluids the child drinks 1–2 hours before bed.
  - Trying potty/urination training pants for the child.
  - Giving them some time—till then use a mattress protector.
- Avoid punishing or teasing child.
- Avoid foods high in sugar and also carbonated and caffeinated beverages.
- Write the episodes down to know the frequency.
- Celebrate successes if the episodes are less or have stopped.

SOILING

ABOUT SOILING

In 1926, Weissenberg was the first person to introduce the term 'encopresis', derived from the Greek word *kopros*, meaning stool. This term was used to describe cases of functional or psychological soiling. In contrast, he reserved the term 'faecal incontinence' for situations involving organic or physiological factors that led to a loss of bowel control.[12]

There are cultural factors that dictate the age by which a child should attain bowel control. Most children in urban societies have erratic faecal continence in the first two years, with the rates declining between ages 3 and 7 as they grow up. For the most part, parents often bring specially-abled or learning-disabled children for treatment due to psychosocial concerns—not just as medical problems.

Learning to void or control one's urinary urge is not as easy as it is perceived by certain parents. Problems of continence are common in childhood. Instead of understanding a child's psychology, putting pressure on the child causes a great deal of anguish and trouble to both child and parents, or the babysitter. Though the control of excreta is physiological, requiring the proper functioning of the autonomic nervous and muscular systems of the urinary bladder and gut, children need to be taught the value of continence.

In addition, they need to have sufficient motivational urge and responsibility to follow the expectations of parents, caregivers and also themselves.

In 2013, a 28-year-old woman residing in Chembur, India, underwent surgery to address an unusually large faecal mass, described as being the size of a football, following an astonishing 45 days without bowel movement.[13]

INCIDENCE

According to the *New Indian Journal of Pediatrics*, constipation ranks among the top ten most-common conditions in paediatrics, affecting about 3 per cent of patients in a general paediatric outpatient department and 20–25 per cent in specialty clinics. Among these cases, 1.3–5 per cent are associated with encopresis, a distressing and anxiety-inducing problem for both the child and the parents.[14]

FACTS BEHIND IT

- Chronic constipation (defined as inability to release stools from the bowels) is the primary cause of soiling.
- The reasons can be biological or accidental soiling.
- Other reasons can be stress, dehydration and pain caused by a sore in or near the anus.

CAUSES

- Long-term constipation
- Slow metabolism
- Fewer bowel movements
- Trauma
- Emotional causes include:
  Limited access to a toilet or shyness over its use or stressful life events, chronic constipation or retention could be a likely outcome of sexual abuse.
- Physical causes include:
  Diarrhoea, constipation or weakening of anal muscles or intestinal nerves
- Retentive soiling causes include:
  Emotional underpinnings, lack of sensitivity to rectal sensation and distension, or abnormal contraction of the voluntary muscles of the pelvis during defecation
- It is not clear whether physiological difficulties are present before symptoms occur in retentive soiling. In addition, the role of genetics or heredity has not been established so far.
- Faecal incontinence may occur due to a persistent leak of fluid faeces. This may emerge because of a physical disorder involving structural or functional difficulties in the gut—leakage of semisolid faeces into the undergarments.
- Some children may place fully formed stools in unusual or inappropriate places. This may again have a psychological or psychiatric trigger.
- Familial stress during infancy and preschool years appears to be a potential contributory trigger for retentive soiling in some children. The role of low intelligence or developmental delays in language comprehension can lead to retentive soiling.

SYMPTOMS

- Involuntary passage of stools
- Leakage of stool or liquid stool on innerwear
- Long-term accumulation of stools causing soreness of anus
- Avoiding bowel movements purposely

Types of soiling:

- Primary incontinence: This refers to patterns occurring in the absence of the child being continent.
- Secondary incontinence: This refers to patterns occurring in a child who was previously continent.

COMPLICATIONS

- Complications may result as a consequence of negative response to open bowels in apprehension of additional physical attack, or due to fear of anal injury.
- Repetitive symptoms can lead to chronic dilation of the rectum.
- Behavioural and emotional problems, or resistance to psychological and medical treatment.
- Parents should relook at basic toilet training techniques and reinforce toilet behaviours without being rude or abusive. Regular and predictable toilet habits with rewards is often a useful method.

HEALING WITH HOMEOPATHY

Soiling	**Homeopathic Remedy**
Involuntary passage of loose, watery stools while passing flatus	*Aloe socotrina*

Soiling	**Homeopathic Remedy**
Offensive smelling, green stool with marked urgency to pass stool	*Podophyllum peltatum*
Constipation with hardness of stools	*Causticum*
During urination or sleep due to a weak anal sphincter	*Hyoscyamus niger*
While laughing, sneezing or passing flatus	*Sulphur*
Excessive flatulence and bloating	*China officinalis*
Suppressed emotions	*Staphysagria*

Dose: 30C pills twice a day, until symptoms subside.
Please consult your doctor before starting medication.

TREATMENT

The treatment for wetting, soiling, faecal incontinence and retentive soiling should be preceded by a thorough examination to rule out any physical disease of the gut. In addition, psychological or behavioural treatment is required alongside professional homeopathic treatment.

CASE STUDY

Kristin, a well-dressed and polite 10-year-old boy with neatly styled hair and matching sneakers, visited the clinic with his father. A little hesitantly, Kristin's father detailed Kristin's long-standing struggle with constipation and soiling, which had begun after his parents' divorce. The family had earlier hoped that Kristin would eventually outgrow these distressing and disruptive episodes. But over the past four years, Kristin had been experiencing soiling episodes daily, without any sensation of urge or leakage. His paediatrician had recommended only laxatives, which did not provide a lasting solution. Recognising the emotional and psychological aspects of his condition, the homeopathic remedy *Staphysagria* was prescribed to address the suppressed emotions, past traumatic events and the mental struggles he was facing. This treatment helped Kristin successfully overcome his episodes, providing relief and alleviating his father's distress.

SELF-HELP

- Bowel training: adjust child's position to ensure easy passage of stools.
- Maintain a toilet timetable or routine.
- Help the child to overcome this situation.
- Don't blame, criticise or punish the child.
- Offer unconditional love and support to the child.
- Help the child with exercises to strengthen the pelvic floor muscles. Start by tightening the pelvic floor muscles for three seconds, then relaxing for three seconds. Try to repeat this ten times a day.

NAIL BITING

ABOUT NAIL BITING

Nail biting is also known as onychophagy or onychophagia. It is a compulsive habit of biting one's fingernails. The first recorded instance of nail biting is attributed to the Stoic philosopher Cleanthes of Assos, who lived between 330 BC and 230 BC.[15]

INCIDENCE

- Nail biting is a common habit. It often presents as soon as the child learns to control movements of the hands.

- The habit tends to affect girls more than boys but they can exist in both sexes. This can bring in a sense of guilt, shame and ridicule in some children.
- According to studies, up to 40 per cent teenagers and 30 per cent adults have a habit of nail biting which can become so severe that 40 per cent of them damage their teeth due to it.[16]

CAUSES

Nail biting is often a result of a child's outlook towards his or her parents. When such a feeling is curbed, it may lead to gross conflict. The result is that the child starts biting nails with a vengeance to overcome a sense of failure, shame, hostility and also resentment. Nail biting is not confined to growing children. It can affect adults too as a fallout of an earlier attempt at suicide or sexual gratification.

Nail biting also plays the role of an outlet, as a means to get rid of tension or anxiety. An exciting cricket match or a suspense movie, for example, can lead to a binge of 'nail biting'.

Research suggests that inadequate or unsatisfactory breastfeeding may also be one of the causative factors for the development of the habit, aside from environmental influences, lullabies or storytelling by a loving adult.

Nail biting is an active process; thumb- and finger-sucking are passive. The latter affects nearly all babies in the first year of life.

Nail biting may also sometimes affect children who have no emotional problems, although it may, like thumb- and finger-sucking, provide the individual a channel to escape from emotional stress. When the habits extend beyond age 3–4, they can lead to baby talk, bedwetting and worm infection.

Children, who are prone to worm infestations, should be cajoled to giving up the habit. Otherwise, getting rid of worms can be extremely difficult.

SYMPTOMS

- Distressful feelings of unease or tension prior to biting
- Feelings of relief or even pleasure after biting
- Feelings of shame, embarrassment, anxiety or guilt, often related to the appearance of physical damage to the skin and nails caused by biting
- Sensations such as itching, tingling or pain that causes the person to bite
- Damage to the tissues around fingers and cuticles

COMPLICATIONS

- Dental problems and finger necrosis
- Damage to the skin around the nail, increasing the risk of infection
- Increase the risk of colds, worms and other infections by spreading germs from your fingers to the mouth

HEALING WITH HOMEOPATHY

Nail Biting	**Homeopathic Remedy**
Children who have an irritable nature	*Cina maritima*
Nervous and anxious personalities with a marked fear of death	*Arsenicum album*
Sad and depressed personalities	*Natrum muriaticum*
Tend to bite their nails until they start to bleed	*Arum triphyllum*
Anxiety	*Aconite napellus*

Nail Biting	Homeopathic Remedy
Mood changes	*Medorrhinum*
Low confidence, poor self-esteem and have fear of appearing in the public	*Lycopodium clavatum*
Rough, brittle and yellow nails with ulcers	*Silicea*

Dose: 30C pills twice a day, until symptoms subside.
Please consult your doctor before starting medication.

CASE STUDY

A 5-year-old boy was brought to the Department of Pedodontics by his parents for his persistent habit of biting his fingernails and toenails. This had been going on since he was 9 months old. The visible damage to his nails attested to this habit. Despite all sorts of attempts, he continued his habit. He also had frequent episodes of stomach ache due to worm infestations. The boy had a stubborn, irritable nature and nail biting seemed to be his primary activity. Recognising the connection between his nervousness, irritability, sleeplessness and susceptibility to worm infestations, the homeopathic remedy *Cina maritima* was prescribed. Gradually, *Cina* helped to alleviate his irritability and nail-biting tendencies. Subsequent follow-up appointments showed a reduction in his stubbornness as well, indicating a positive outcome from the treatment.

SELF-HELP

- Avoid factors that trigger nail biting.
- Keep nails neatly trimmed.
- Occupy hands or mouth with alternate activities.
- Apply a bitter tasting lacquer to nails to discourage biting.
- Distract yourself with a stress ball.

THUMB- AND FINGER-SUCKING

ABOUT THUMB- AND FINGER-SUCKING

It is reported that approximately 1 in 10 adults may engage in thumb-sucking at some point in their lives. A few individuals suck their thumb since childhood, while others may adopt it to alleviate anxiety or stress.[17]

INCIDENCE

According to the American Academy of Pediatrics, 70–90 per cent of children engage in thumb-sucking behaviour. Interestingly, thumb-sucking can begin even before birth, as some babies exhibit this reflex in the womb itself.[18]

CAUSES

- Out of habit
- Due to hunger
- Due to boredom or stress

SYMPTOMS

- Habit of putting the thumb in the mouth for comfort or to relieve stress

COMPLICATIONS

- Dental malocclusion—misalignment of the teeth
- Persistent, vigorous thumb-sucking can cause not just misalignment of the child's permanent teeth but also affect the jaw or the shape and roof of the mouth
- Speech impediment

RESEARCH

A study published in the *British Homeopathic Journal* examined the effects of homeopathic treatment on children diagnosed with ADHD. In this study, the children were divided into two groups: one group received homeopathic treatment, while the other group was given a placebo for a period of ten days. The behaviour of the children was assessed by both their parents and teachers. The results of the study revealed that the children who received homeopathic medicines demonstrated a significant reduction in behaviour within just ten days.[19]

HEALING WITH HOMEOPATHY

Calcarea carbonicum 30C, 4 pills taken twice a day, helps children who have the problem of thumb- and finger-sucking. To be taken until symptoms subside. Please consult your doctor before starting medication.

CASE STUDY

Three-year-old Rani had been sucking her thumb since she was only 20 days old and despite her parents' persistent efforts to break the habit, it endured. Rani, a plump and seemingly lethargic child, consistently sought the presence of her parents, often accompanied by her indulgent brother. Rani's parents tried various activities to keep her hands occupied, but during her free time, she would revert to thumb-sucking. Her father observed that she covered her thumb with her other hand, seemingly to conceal the behaviour. Rani was prescribed *Calcarea carbonicum* based on her sluggishness, overweight and constant need for parental support. After a few doses, the frequency of her thumb-sucking diminished, and she began to enjoy engaging in various games which she had previously overlooked.

SELF-HELP

- Try using thumb puppets or thumbsters for the child to avoid sucking.
- Parents can help calm their child in extreme situations which lead to thumb-sucking.
- Create a chart to track child behaviour and reward them when reduction of thumb-sucking is observed.
- Avoid criticising and admonishing the child for thumb-sucking.

EMOTIONAL DISORDERS IN TEENS

HAIR-TWIRLING

FACTS BEHIND IT

Hair-twirling is considered part of a group of habits known as fidgets, which includes thumb-sucking. In a similar way to thumb-sucking, a child may twirl their hair to soothe themselves, to calm anxiety, to deal with boredom or to wind down before sleep.

CAUSES

- Stress and anxiety
- Having upsetting thoughts or impulses that occur repeatedly

SYMPTOMS

- Hair-twirling first appears in early childhood as a forerunner to hair-pulling (trichotillomania).
- It may be accompanied with or without hair loss.
- Most children give up the habit, once they grow up—more so, with professional homeopathic treatment.

COMPLICATIONS

- Excessive twirling or pulling of hair can result in hair loss or bald patches.
- Follicle damage
- Dangerous compulsive behaviours
- When hair-twirling extends to adulthood, it is often difficult to break.

RESEARCH

Homeopathy treats people suffering from hair-twirling and improves the body's response to stress and anxiety. This, in turn, helps in controlling the urge to pull out one's hair or twirl it. Since the treatment addresses the root cause of the problem, it reduces the chances of recurrence.

HEALING WITH HOMEOPATHY

For hair-twirling and pulling of hair, *Kalium phosphoricum* is a useful remedy.

The dose is 30C pills twice a day, until symptoms subside. Please consult your doctor before starting medication.

CASE STUDY

A 43-year-old woman suffered from a traumatic experience and after that she developed a long-standing habit of twirling and occasionally pulling her hair. This behaviour had been going on for approximately 27 years (from the time she was 16) and had been progressively increasing in severity. This habit began during her high school years, initially with hair-twirling and later escalating to hair-pulling. During this time, she managed to hide any bald spots that developed due to the hair-pulling. Before going out, she would use an eye pencil to cover the bald spots, and if anyone inquired, she attributed it to hair loss caused by a vitamin deficiency. Over time, her hair loss became too extensive to conceal. She resorted to wearing a bandana when going out and even started wearing it at home, hoping that this would help her pull out less hair. Finally, with her husband's support, she decided to seek treatment. She was prescribed *Kalium phosphoricum*, a remedy known for its calming effect on the nerves. After 2–3 months, she reported substantial improvement in both her mental and physical condition. Her bald spots showed positive signs of hair regrowth, and she was highly motivated to continue with the treatment. As a result, she no longer felt the need to use a bandana.

SELF-HELP

- Keep on changing the hairstyle, don't stick to one particular partition.
- Keeping shorter hair can help as the child may find it too rough to handle and hence not soothing.
- Fidget devices can provide distraction and relief that a fidgety child looks for.
- Brush the hair instead of twirling.
- Do something constructive instead of sitting idle.
- Reward and appreciate if the child does not twirl for a longer time.

BOREDOM

> Boredom doesn't exist where creativity lives.
>
> —Unknown

ABOUT BOREDOM

'Boredom' was first officially recognised as a word in 1852, coinciding with the publication of Charles Dickens's complex and occasionally tedious serial *Bleak House*. Roman philosopher Seneca likened boredom to a form of nausea, emphasising its unpleasant nature, while Greek historian Plutarch mentioned that Pyrrhus, known for the 'pyrrhic victory', experienced profound boredom during his retirement. These historical references suggest that boredom has been a part of human experience for centuries.[20]

INCIDENCE

A comprehensive psychosocial study was conducted in the United States to investigate the prevalence of high boredom. The research was done on a nationally representative samples of 8th and 10th graders, comprising 21,173 participants. The study stated that roughly 20 per cent of adolescents reported experiencing high levels of boredom.[21]

According to the Mondelez International and The Harris Poll, 8 out of 10 Indians have started snacking to overcome their boredom, which is well above the global level.[22]

A study conducted by Carnegie Mellon University revealed that 63 per cent of American adults encounter boredom at least once every 10 days. The study also said that boredom is more prevalent in men, young individuals, those who are unmarried and those with lower income levels.[23]

Interestingly, a study conducted by psychologists at the University of Virginia found that around two-thirds of men and a quarter of women would opt to self-administer electric shocks to themselves rather than be left alone in an empty room for a mere 15 minutes. This suggests a strong aversion that some people have toward boredom, to the extent that they would choose a painful experience as a means of alleviating it.[24]

FACTS BEHIND IT

According to a research study, individuals who respond more negatively to boredom might exhibit distinct brain wave patterns before actually experiencing boredom. The study says that people who frequently grapple with boredom are more likely to suffer from poor mental health with heightened risk of conditions like anxiety and depression.[25]

CAUSES

- Inadequate rest
- Malnutrition
- Fear of making a mistake
- Repetition of an activity for too much time
- Feeling unable to try new approaches to the activity

SYMPTOMS

- Chronic feeling of emptiness
- Sense of frustration with idleness
- Limited attention span

- Lack of interest in regular work and activities
- Apathetic
- Fatigued
- Nervous
- Jittery

COMPLICATIONS

- Depression and anxiety
- Anger
- Academic failure
- Poor work performance
- Loneliness
- Isolation
- Individuals with ADHD get bored faster and may have more difficulty in concentrating than others

HEALING WITH HOMEOPATHY

Boredom	**Homeopathic Remedy**
Weak memory and lack of concentration and confidence; mentally and physically weak child. They take a long time to comprehend a topic, keep reading the topic again and again; child's height is less than their age; they are very shy, with few friends	*Baryta carbonicum*
Child is very nervous and irritable with loss of memory, slightest labour seems a heavy task, is shy, with changeable moods	*Kalium phosphoricum*
Child make mistakes in spellings and names when writing; sometimes when they speak to someone, repeatedly lose the thread of a conversation because they forget the word	*Medorrhinum*

Boredom	Homeopathic Remedy
A serious loss of memory; cannot talk without help from others; they cannot even start a conversation without support	*Kalium bromatum*
Cannot remember what was taught; lack of interest in studies, inability to digest milk	*Aethusa cynapium*
Fat, chubby children who grow rapidly; forgetful and confused, always lazy and sleepy	*Calcarea carbonicum*
Child is fearful, forgetful, lack of concentration	*Phosphorus*
Feel tired and drained very soon during studies; child cannot bear mental exertion, inability to think and sleeplessness	*Magnesium phosphoricum*
Anaemic child; there are ill effects of anger, fright and grief	*Natrum muriaticum*
Lack of fear in the child, has performance anxiety and examination phobia	*Gelsemium sempervirens*

Dose: 30C pills, twice a day until symptoms subside.
Please consult your doctor before starting medication.

CASE STUDY

Riya's mother expressed her concerns about her daughter, 'I am truly stressed about my daughter's behaviour. I am a housewife, and my husband is overseas, so I live with my in-laws. During the pandemic, staying at home led Riya to watch TV and use the computer and mobile phone all the time. She lost interest in writing or learning, as her school provided daily assignments. She couldn't sit in one place for even a few minutes, not even when watching TV. I don't know how to handle her.' Additionally, Riya had difficulty remembering what she was taught, and she had developed a strong aversion to milk. The homeopathic remedy *Aethusa cynapium* was advised for Riya, based on the specific symptom of milk intolerance, with the expectation of addressing both her physical and mental behaviour. After receiving the prescribed doses, Riya began to recite poems and showed interest in sharing her school experiences with her mother. Gradually, her milk intolerance also reduced, indicating positive progress in both her behaviour and physical condition.

SELF-HELP

- Keep a record of the circumstances in which the child becomes bored.
- Note the time of day, place and activities, so that those circumstances can be avoided.
- Break larger tasks into smaller ones, and plan breaks or rewards at key milestones.
- Avoid showing impatience or anxiety when dealing with the child.
- Help the child identify their emotions.

BULLYING

> Bullies only have power if you let them.
>
> —Aaron Korsh

ABOUT BULLYING

In the mid-1970s, Dan Olweus, a research professor of psychology, conducted an in-depth study on bullying among students, employing his unique research methods. He then pioneered the creation of the Olweus Bullying Prevention Programme. Olweus's work made a significant contribution to addressing the problem of bullying and promoting a safer and more respectful atmosphere in schools. This programme also had a profound impact on reducing school violence and reinstating a sense of safety in educational environments.[26]

INCIDENCE

A 2022 report by the cyber security firm McAfee revealed alarming statistics. Around 85 per cent of Indian children have experienced cyberbullying, making it the highest prevalence globally. Indian children also reported being victims of cyberbullying and engaging in cyberbullying behaviour at rates significantly higher than the global average. More than 1 in 3 children reported facing issues such as cyber racism, sexual harassment and threats of physical harm as early as the age of 10.[27]

CAUSES

The causes of bullying are many, but a few are common.

Being Bullied	**The One Who Bullies**
• Physical disability • Stunted height • Stammering • Racial differences • Inappropriate weight	• Expression of anger • When something unrelated becomes the focal point of frustration • Poor upbringing • Someone who bullies others might have experienced bullying themselves • Seeing violent games or movies • Bullies are often lonely • Frustration or envy

SYMPTOMS

Being Bullied	**The One Who Bullies**
Emotional and behavioural signs of being bullied: • Change in sleep and eating patterns • Mood swings • Frequent tears or anger • Stammering • Unreasonably aggressive • Refuses to talk about what is wrong • Sibling rivalry • Loses money or starts stealing	Emotional and behavioural signs of bullying others: • Likes violence • Controls and dominates others • Hot-tempered, impulsive and gets easily frustrated • Breaks rules often
Physical signs of being bullied: • Unexplained bruises, cuts, scratches • Frequent missing or damaged belongings or clothes • Always hungry	Physical signs of bullying others: • Aggressive towards parents, teachers • Those who bully tend to be physically stronger than their peers
School-related signs of being bullied: • Refusal to attend school • Change of route to school • Poor academic grades	School-related signs of bullying others: • Frequent visits to principal's office
Other signs of being bullied: • Often alone; a loner • Excluded from peer group • Always appearing frightened in any new situation • Damaged or missing possessions with no explanation	Other signs of bullying others: • Girl bullies want to win at all costs • Dramatic in nature • Over-aggressive • Have unexplained extra money or new belongings

COMPLICATIONS

- A desire for isolation
- Lack of motivation
- Stammering
- Bedwetting
- Self-harming behaviour or suicide attempts

HEALING WITH HOMEOPATHY

Bullying	**Homeopathic Remedy**
In nervous children and those who are scared of being left alone or left with strangers	*Baryta carbonicum*
Excessively nervous children who are easily frightened by the slightest noise	*Borax*
Children who have difficulty in learning at school, but they usually do their homework scrupulously	*Arsenicum album*
Children who are anxious before school. They are like angels at school and devils at home.	*Lycopodium clavatum*
Children who suffer from anticipatory anxiety before examination	*Gelsemium sempervirens*
Children who suffer from bad events in the past	*Natrum muriaticum*
Complaints from a recent disturbing event	*Ignatia amara*

Dose: 30C pills, twice a day until symptoms subside.
Please consult your doctor before starting medication.

CASE STUDY

Vikti, a 15-year-old girl, moved to a new school. In her first week, she encountered Bertha in the cafeteria, who proceeded to insult and criticise Vikti's clothes, hairstyle and appearance. Bertha even encouraged others to join in these hurtful comments. Vikti, deeply affected by this negative experience, began avoiding the cafeteria and confided in her mother that Bertha had abused her. This incident had such a profound emotional impact on Vikti that she resorted to self-harm, inflicting multiple cuts on her hands and knees. She withdrew from social activities, became increasingly isolated and developed disordered eating habits, spending most of her day in bed. Distressed with all this, Vikti's parents sought counselling and homeopathic treatment for her. She was prescribed the homeopathic remedy *Ignatia amara* for addressing emotional turmoil following the traumatic events. After two follow-up sessions, Vikti showed improvement in her mental symptoms. However, she still refused to go to school. Her parents remained patient and optimistic, believing that with regular follow-up treatments, Vikti would eventually feel comfortable about returning to school. After three months of treatment, there was a positive turnaround, and Vikti resumed attending school. This progress highlights the effectiveness of both counselling and homeopathic treatment in helping Vikti recover and regain her confidence.

SELF-HELP

- Having a good relationship with the child is the first step to resolving the problem.
- Give comfort to the child and get him or her to describe what happened during the incident.
- Pamper the child.
- Don't let the child feel low.
- Make him or her understand that everything will eventually pass by.

- Give options to the child of texting or writing a letter or talking on the phone to explain the incident if he or she is not comfortable about expressing everything face-to-face.
- Make them understand the cons of posting every update of theirs on social media.
- Check that their web surfing is age-appropriate.
- Always make sure that the child saves the evidence of the incident to show the guardian or the teacher.

DISAPPOINTMENT IN LOVE

INCIDENCE

Based on statistics released by the National Crime Records Bureau (NCRB), India witnessed a heartbreaking total of 135,445 suicides in 2012. A closer examination of these statistics reveals the daily toll, with 242 men and 129 women taking their own lives every day. On average, 15 suicides occur each hour, amounting to a total of 371 suicides daily.[28]

CAUSES

- Unrealistic standards
- Inability to express feelings
- Comparing their relationships with others' relationships
- Seeing the partner as inferior
- Holding on to the past problems or actions by the partner
- Lack of trust
- Lack of respect
- Either partner does not forgive or forget

SYMPTOMS

- Anger and frustration
- Crying and sadness
- Insomnia
- Loss of interest in day-to-day activities
- Feelings of hopelessness or helplessness
- Thoughts of death or suicide

COMPLICATIONS

- Depression
- Trouble thinking clearly or making decisions
- Slow moving or talking
- Thoughts of death
- Suicide

RESEARCH

According to the American Psychological Association, the divorce rate in the United States varies based on the order of marriage. Approximately 40–50 per cent of first marriages end in divorce. The divorce rate for second marriages is even higher, with approximately 60–67 per cent of second marriages ending in divorce.[29]

HEALING WITH HOMEOPATHY

Disappointment in Love	**Homeopathic Remedy**
Crying, sobbing, sleeplessness, with desire to stay alone, constant state of deep thought, dwells on past events	*Ignatia amara*
Inconsolable and prolonged weeping spells; mind occupied by thoughts of the unpleasant episode that triggers the grief	*Natrum muriaticum*

Disappointment in Love	**Homeopathic Remedy**
Suicidal thoughts	*Aurum metallicum*
Loss of interest in life or the outside world; does not wish to go out; doesn't talk to anyone	*Phosphoricum acidum*

Dose: 30C pills, twice a day until symptoms subside.
Please consult your doctor before starting medication.

SELF-HELP

- Don't dwell on past events
- Continuous thinking of the past can slow down the progress of recovery from mental illnesses
- Try navigating through negative situation, seeking solutions
- Share your thoughts and feelings openly and fully with your peers, fostering deeper connections and understanding
- Avoid being harsh on yourself—the situation eventually changes and improves with time
- Don't let social media influence have a negative impact over your life

EMOTIONAL DISORDERS IN OLD AGE

> What makes old age so sad is not that our joys but that our hopes then cease.
>
> —Jean Paul

DEPRESSION

ABOUT DEPRESSION

In the 19th century, German psychiatrist Emil Kraepelin played a significant role in the evolution of psychiatric terminology. He began using the term 'depressive states' to describe various forms of melancholia, primarily because of the characteristic low mood that characterises these conditions.[30]

Depression was known in the second millennium BC in Mesopotamia. People of that time believed that it was caused by a demonic possession and accordingly it was managed by priests rather than medical professionals.

Due to this belief, treatments often included harsh methods such as beatings, physical restraints and starvation, all intended to drive out the demons supposedly causing the condition.[31]

INCIDENCE

The prevalence of depression among the elderly population in India is reported to be at 34.4 per cent, according to a study published in BMC Public Health.[32]

CAUSES

- Being single, divorced or widowed
- Lack of a supportive social network
- Stressful life events
- Transitioning from work to retirement
- Financial hardships
- Chronic medical conditions
- Dependence on others, whether through being hospitalised or needing home healthcare

- Disability
- Past suicidal attempts
- Substance abuse

SYMPTOMS

- Feeling of tiredness
- Altered sleep patterns
- Being grumpy or irritable
- Struggle focusing on anything
- Feeling of worthlessness
- Do not enjoy activities they used to
- Thoughts to leave house
- Suicidal thoughts

COMPLICATIONS

- Decreased mobility in older adults often stems from factors like muscle weakness, joint issues and balance problems, impacting their ability to move freely.
- Isolation.
- The limitations of mobility in older adults can sometimes serve as a reminder of their mortality, prompting reflection on life's changes and challenges.
- As depression advances, the individual seems to expect failure at every step.
- They think there is no happiness in life.
- Suicidal thoughts

RESEARCH

Anxiety and depression are among the most frequently treated conditions by homeopaths. A study was conducted at a university hospital outpatient clinic that involved 6,544 patients who used homeopathy as a part of their treatment. Of these, 205 patients were specifically treated for depression, and a noteworthy finding was that as many as 71 per cent of these patients showed improvement. This research provides confirmation of the positive outcomes and experiences in treating individuals with depression through homeopathy.[33]

HEALING WITH HOMEOPATHY

Depression	**Homeopathic Remedy**
Excessive worriers who are particularly obsessed about their health	*Arsenicum album*
Workaholics with a tendency to feel worthlessness, despair and suicidal thoughts after a failure	*Aurum metallicum*
Reliable and hard-working individuals who become overwhelmed by physical illness	*Calcarea carbonica*
Depressed after a loss or when grieving; forgetful, regularly crying and mental dullness	*Causticum*
Active and conversational during good times; however, they feel low and upset during episodes of depression	*Cimicifuga racemosa*
Sensitive people who tend to suppress disappointment or grief	*Ignatia amara*
Jealousy, suspicion or repressed feelings, menopausal depression	*Lachesis muta*
Depressed from disappointment of any kind	*Natrum carbonicum*
Long standing grief with suppression of emotions	*Natrum muriaticum*
Tearful and sad when depressed, depression occurs in conjunction with menopause, menstrual periods or puberty.	*Pulsatilla nigricans*

Depression	**Homeopathic Remedy**
Challenging to manage and overcome their loved ones needs, feelings etc., better after crying and they prefer not to be consoled	*Sepia officinalis*
Depression caused by shame, resentment, suppressed emotions, and hurt feelings	*Staphysagria*

Dose: *Kalium phosphoricum* 6X, two tablets thrice a day helps those who suffer from depression after prolonged periods of emotional stress or excitement.

Please consult your doctor before starting medication.

CASE STUDY

Dhanvantari, a 60-year-old woman, was brought to the clinic by her husband, who was concerned about her struggle with depression, which had been going on for over five years. During this period, she was on anti-depressant medications. She had also become emotionally distant from her husband and their two children. Upon analysis of her case, it was revealed that her depression had emerged following surgery. The surgery involved the removal of her uterus due to a tumour, which had resulted in hormonal imbalances and, subsequently, depression. Based on her emotional state characterised by listless indifference towards her loved ones, along with her hormonal imbalance, the homeopathic remedy *Sepia officinalis* was prescribed for her. After five months of homeopathic treatment, she visited the clinic with her husband, and the positive changes were evident. Her husband confirmed that she had started taking interest in her daily activities and had become more loving and caring towards her family.

SELF-HELP

- Talk openly with peers and family about the situation and the problems faced.
- Facing rather than avoiding distressing or challenging issues promotes growth, resilience and the potential for resolution or understanding.
- Practise laughter therapy.
- Studies have shown that low sodium diets reduce possibility of depression.
- Tryptophan-rich food is considered helpful in reducing depression. The sources include dates, milk, yoghurt, cottage cheese, meat, fish, poultry, sesame, chickpeas, peanuts, soyabeans and soya products.
- Food containing omega-3 fatty acid helps in healthy mental functioning—flaxseeds, wheat germ, linseed, black currants and sesame seeds.
- Avoid alcohol, excess sugar and caffeine.

LOSS OF MEMORY

> We remember their love when they no longer remember.
>
> —Unknown

ABOUT LOSS OF MEMORY

German physician Alois Alzheimer is well known for describing the case of Auguste D., a patient who exhibited profound memory loss and who had unwarranted suspicions regarding her family as well as other psychological issues. Upon conducting an autopsy of Auguste's brain, Alzheimer made a groundbreaking discovery. He observed dramatic shrinkage of the brain and the presence of abnormal deposits in and around the nerve cells. This seminal case provided crucial insights into the medical condition that would later bear Alzheimer's name and paved the way for further research into the disease.[34]

INCIDENCE

According to the 'Dementia India' report published by the Alzheimer's and Related Disorders Society of India, India is home to the second-largest number of individuals globally, suffering from dementia. The report estimates that approximately 4.1 million people in India are living with dementia, and this number is projected to double by the year 2035.[35]

FACTS BEHIND IT

Alzheimer's is triggered by the accumulation of abnormal proteins in the brain. Amyloid forms deposits, creating plaques around cells, while it twists into tangled cells, disrupting normal brain function.

SYMPTOMS

- Confusion of time or place
- Misplacing things
- Losing the ability to retrace steps
- Decreased or poor judgement
- Withdrawal from work and social activities
- Changes in mood and personality
- Forgetting which day it is and remembering it later
- Challenges in planning or solving problems
- Difficulty in completing familiar tasks

COMPLICATIONS

- Diminished quality of life
- Reduced lifespan
- In some cases, lost memories can't be recovered

RESEARCH

According to the journal *Homeopathy*, the homeopathy medicine *Lycopodium clavatum* is beneficial in cases of dementia.[36]

HEALING WITH HOMEOPATHY

Loss of Memory	Homeopathic Remedy
Sudden loss of memory, especially under stress	*Anacardium orientale*
Feeling of floating or unreality, disorientation and confusion with forgetfulness	*Cannabis indica*
Apathy, dullness, slowness and blankness of mind, poor concentration	*Helleborus niger*
Gradual memory loss, confusion and dyslexia; words are misused or misplaced	*Lycopodium clavatum*
Sudden loss of thoughts; absent-minded and dreamy	*Nux moschata*
Forgetfulness and apathy from grief, brooding about the past and future	*Phosphoricum acidum*
Absent-minded and forgetful of words; makes mistakes in writing or speaking	*Sulphur*

CASE STUDY

Lata, a 63-year-old woman, sought medical advice due to memory loss issues after her retirement. Her spouse had noticed a decline in her cognitive skills, with difficulties in processing information and carrying out instructions. She had also demonstrated signs of not being able to perform routine tasks like turning off the stove. Lata had also ceased driving a motor vehicle approximately six months prior to seeking help. Her medical history included vitamin D deficiency. During the case analysis, Lata revealed that she was dealing with significant emotional stress due to her son's departure from the house after his marriage. This situation had caused her constant worry and disappointment. In response to her emotional state, she was prescribed *Anacardium orientale*. In the subsequent follow-up sessions, her husband reported remarkable improvements. Lata's appetite increased, her cognitive responses improved, and she was better able to remember and execute instructions, indicating a good progress in her overall well-being.

SELF-HELP

- Don't panic—staying calm is the key.
- Maintain a to-do list or a checklist for important tasks of the day.
- Emergency phone numbers should be kept handy.
- Use of sticky notes around the house can help to ease the anxiety.
- Avoid staying alone; always ensure someone's company.
- Sleep affects memory consolidation; a minimum of eight hours sleep is recommended.

9

Lack of Confidence

> If you don't ask, the answer is always 'no'.
>
> —Nora Roberts

INCIDENCE

Low self-esteem took centre stage in an open seminar and panel discussion organised by the Association of Counsellors and Psychotherapists of Nagpur (ACPN). It was estimated 90 per cent of the people were affected by low self-esteem.[1]

CAUSES

- Impaired brain chemicals
- Impaired good-mood hormone
- Hormonal imbalances
- Early childhood trauma
- Situational depression due to sad incidents

SYMPTOMS

- Lack of control over relationships, opinions, work, studies, and so on
- Negative comparisons with others
- Worry and self-doubt
- Trouble accepting positive feedback
- Negative self-talk
- Fear of failure
- Trying to please others

COMPLICATIONS

- Feelings of sadness
- Depression
- Anxiety
- Anger
- Shame
- Guilt

HEALING WITH HOMEOPATHY

Lack of Confidence	**Homeopathic Remedy**
Self-criticising nature	*Aurum metallicum*
Lawyers and professionals who are successful but lack confidence	*Lycopodium clavatum*
Deep insults in the past	*Staphysagria*
Timid	*Silicea*
Anxiety	*Argentum nitricum*
Stunted development and shy with strangers	*Baryta carbonicum*
A fear of examinations, dulling of the memory	*Anacardium orientale*

Dose: 30C pills, twice a day until symptoms subside.
Please consult your doctor before starting medication.

CASE STUDY

Rafiq Khan, a 15-year-old boy, had been experiencing stomach aches for the past three months. He never spoke about his discomfort himself but relied on his mother to express his issues. His mother said that Rafiq lacked confidence, despite his good academic performance. He was always uncertain about his exam performance and hesitated to participate in discussions with friends or venture out on his own. This led him to become introverted. The presence of his high-achieving elder brother, who often encouraged him to compete and consistently win, further eroded Rafiq's self-confidence. Rafiq was prescribed *Silicea* to strengthen the mind. After a month, there was noticeable improvement and a significant boost in Rafiq's confidence and independence.

SELF-HELP

- Talk to someone trustworthy
- Take counselling sessions
- Share the struggles with someone who can offer unconditional support
- Avoid negative thoughts

10

Loneliness

> The most terrible poverty is loneliness, and the feeling of being unloved.
>
> —Mother Teresa

ABOUT LONELINESS

In 1950, David Riesman published the book *The Lonely Crowd*—at a time when only 9 per cent of households were made up of single individuals. Nearly a decade later, in 1959, psychiatry recognised the concept of loneliness in a subtle essay by the German analyst Frieda Fromm-Reichmann.[1]

INCIDENCE

Research based on the first wave (2017–2018) of the Longitudinal Ageing Study in India (LASI) revealed that 20.5 per cent of adults aged 45 and above in India reported experiencing moderate loneliness, and 13.3 per cent reported severe loneliness.[2]

FACTS BEHIND IT

The American Heart Association highlighted that individuals who lead isolated lives face a 50 per cent higher risk of early death, and isolation can increase the risk of stroke and coronary artery disease by 32 per cent.[3]

CAUSES

- Change of school or jobs
- Work from home
- Move to a new city
- End of a relationship

SYMPTOMS

- Decreased energy
- Feeling foggy or unable to focus
- Feelings of self-doubt, hopelessness or worthlessness
- Tendency to fall sick frequently
- Cravings for physical warmth, such as hot drinks, baths or cosy clothes and blankets

COMPLICATIONS

- Alcohol and drug abuse
- Altered brain function
- Alzheimer's disease progression
- Unsocial or antisocial behaviour
- Cardiovascular disease and stroke
- Decreased memory and learning
- Depression and suicide

- Increased stress levels
- Poor decision-making

RESEARCH

The UN called for extra action to protect mental health; due to the COVID-19 pandemic, higher rates of suicide were observed, due to mental health problems or substance abuse. Homeopathic treatment has a long and successful track record of supporting people with mental health difficulties without any side effects.[4]

HEALING WITH HOMEOPATHY

Loneliness	**Homeopathic Remedy**
Due to a recent sad event	*Ignatia amara*
Chronic depression with isolating oneself and avoid going out	*Natrum muriaticum*
Major depression with suicidal thoughts	*Aurum metallicum*
Desires solitude and often sits quietly alone	*Sepia officinalis*

Dose: 30C pills, twice a day until symptoms subside.
Please consult your doctor before starting medication.

CASE STUDY

Ruthu became widow at 37 when she was 7 months pregnant. The couple had been enjoying life travelling wherever they fancied, and were expecting a baby without any worries. When her husband collapsed in bed, Ruthu felt guilty about not being able to turn him over due to her pregnancy. She stayed with his family, but loneliness and grief overwhelmed her, and she often locked herself in, crying in bed. Only close friends and family understood her pain. Ruthu couldn't bear to leave the house that reminded her of her late husband. She was prescribed homeopathic medicine *Ignatia amara* for her grief, which greatly improved her emotional state.

SELF-HELP

- Try focusing on positive thoughts.
- Talk to people who share similar attitudes, interests and values with you.
- Keep control over the time you spend online and what you surf.
- Understand that ups and downs in life need to be taken positively.
- Do not acquire addictions and take extreme steps.
- Socialise more, try making new friends and join yoga, dance or other activity classes.
- Overcome the situation, rather than living in it.
- Letting go is required.
- Try seeking professional counselling.

11

Mood Swings

> Moods never take permission before they change.

Fluctuating moods are common as we pass through life and learn to surmount its upheavals. Emotional insecurity is often found more commonly among women. They are especially vulnerable as they go through painful phases during puberty, pregnancy and menopause. People's moods can change rapidly—hatred, overbearing love, sudden bursts of communication and equally understandable periods of complete silence. Mood fluctuations can at times even turn a person violent. When the fluctuations are severe, they lead to what is medically called manic depressive psychosis. When this happens too often, it sets off an unpredictable, tense atmosphere. Family members are often at a loss, not knowing how to react to such outbursts. Timely medical help and an understanding of psychological processes often help the individual tide over such stress periods.

In some individuals, moods could vacillate because of a traumatic incident—either a death in the family or disappointment in love or even plain fright. Disturbed childhood experiences could modify a person's behaviour, making it undesirable.

INCIDENCE

According to an article published in *BMJ Open Publishing*, 78 out of 1,000 Indians suffer from mood swings.[1]

According to *Medical News Today*, more than 16.1 million adults in the US experience mood swings, characterised by persistent feelings of sadness and a loss of interest in activities they usually enjoy.[2]

FACTS BEHIND IT

Abnormal level of neurotransmitters may result in mood swings or a mood disorder. Serotonin is one such neurotransmitter that is involved with sleep, moods and emotional states. A slight imbalance of this could result in depression.[3]

CAUSES

- Bipolar disorder
- Sleep deprivation
- Low blood sugar
- Stress
- Certain medications
- Hormones
- Pregnancy
- Premenstrual syndrome
- Menopause
- Dementia
- ADHD

- Thyroid malfunction
- Excess caffeine
- Excess sugar
- Depression

SYMPTOMS

- Anxiety, irritability or agitation
- Boredom
- Confusion
- Difficulty with concentration
- Difficulty with memory, thinking, talking, comprehension, writing or reading
- Excess alcohol consumption
- Hallucinations or delusions
- Poor judgement
- Racing thoughts and rapid speech
- Appetite and weight changes
- Incontinence, weakness or sensory changes

COMPLICATIONS

- Brain damage
- Memory loss
- Attention difficulties
- Impaired judgement
- Coma
- Social isolation
- Suicide or violence

RESEARCH

A study published in *Research in Complementary Medicine* aimed to assess the effects of *Nux vomica* and *Coffea cruda* on the subjective mood of healthy adults. The results showed that the remedies had beneficial effects, with improved mood.[4]

HEALING WITH HOMEOPATHY

Mood Swings	**Homeopathic Remedy**
Alternating moods of depression and cheerfulness	*Sepia officinalis*
Women who tend to get excited and irritable during pregnancy	*Nux vomica*
During menopause, black moods with hot palms and severe headaches	*Lachesis muta*
Women who tend to get nervous and tearful	*Graphites*
Problem of recent origin	*Ignatia amara*
Long-standing emotional problem	*Natrum muriaticum*
Ill effects of suppressed anger, resulting in unstable emotions	*Staphysagria*
Alternate between tears and laughter easily	*Pulsatilla nigricans*

Dose: 30C pills, twice a day until symptoms subside.
Please consult your doctor before starting medication.

CASE STUDY

Sujata, a teenager, sought help for premenstrual tension causing mood swings and emotional instability. Her menstrual history showed irregular cycles with normal flow but frequent stomach upsets. She was prescribed *Pulsatilla nigricans* 200, one dose weekly for a month. This reduced her problems during her menstrual cycle and improved emotional stability. She then continued with a single monthly dose for two months, and her condition improved significantly, bringing relief to her and her family.

SELF-HELP

- Note down the triggers and avoid them.
- Do not shout or harm anyone during the episodes.
- Try calming techniques during the mood swings.
- Take proper sleep to avoid irritation.
- Practise stress management techniques.
- Consult a counsellor if the episodes persist.

12

Stress and How to Manage It

> Stress is caused by being 'here' but wanting to be 'there'.
>
> —Eckhart Tolle

Stress is an inevitable part of life and existence. It is a physical, mental or emotional factor that causes tension in the body or the mind. Stress can be external (from the environment or social situations or as a psychological response) or internal (illness or from a medical procedure). Stress can initiate the fight-or-flight response, a complex reaction of neurologic and endocrinology systems. People having chronic stress or anxiety tend to have persistently raised levels of adrenaline and noradrenaline.

Stress is one of the contributing factors for headaches and migraines, backaches, anxiety, depression and sleep difficulties. Stress can also cause gastrointestinal disorders including ulcers, lower abdominal cramps, colitis, high blood pressure, acid reflux disorder and irritable bowel syndrome. It can also cause loss of libido, cancer, chronic fatigue syndrome, absence of menstruation (amenorrhea), abnormal bleeding, fibroid tumours (in women) and fertility problems in couples. Heart disease and diabetes are also stress-related disorders.

Women are more prone to stress caused by hormonal changes. Stress occurs during puberty, menstrual cycle, pregnancy and menopause, owing to variations in hormone levels. Some women experience changes in their sexual health and develop various sexual dysfunctions such as loss of desire and vaginal dryness because of stress.

Not all stresses are negative. If a person deals with anxiety or stress effectively, stress can help him or her to reach their goals more quickly. This 'good' stress, or 'eustress' motivates and propels people to do well in life and career.

There are, as stress research pioneer Hans Selye propounded, three stages in stressful situations and our response to them:

- An initial period of alarm or physiological arousal.
- A longer phase of resistance, marked by irritability, impatience, anger and fatigue.
- A final stage of exhaustion, represented by physical and emotional imbalance, maladjustment, withdrawal, illness or disease and, in extreme cases, death.

For a holistic treatment, choosing an appropriate homeopathic therapy for reducing stress and anxiety should be supported with counselling, stress management measures, relaxation techniques, taking nutritional supplements such as magnesium and behaviour modification.

ABOUT STRESS

The term 'stress' was coined by Hans Selye, a pioneering researcher in the field of stress physiology, in 1936. He defined it as 'the non-specific response of the body to any demand for change'.[1]

INCIDENCE

According to a report, 24 per cent of Indians are struggling with stress. Current workplace environment and financial uncertainty are the major factors affecting stress levels amongst Indians.[2]

FACTS BEHIND IT

A stressful event triggers the release of hormones, specifically cortisol, by the hypothalamus. These hormones are produced by the adrenal glands and released into the bloodstream. This stress response leads to an increase in blood sugar levels, a more rapid heart rate due to the release of adrenaline and more oxygen being sent to the muscles, which can result in muscle tension.[3]

CAUSES

- Stress has psychological causes and also psychological outcomes.
- It changes the way we perceive the world, our senses, memory, judgement and also behaviour.

SYMPTOMS

- The pupils of the eyes dilate to let in more light and improve the vision.
- Likewise, mental alertness and reaction time are also speeded up.

COMPLICATIONS

- People with severe stress may be subject to frequent colds and infections or allergies. Stress can set off skin conditions such as itching and rashes, including atopic dermatitis (eczema) and psoriasis.
- Prolonged stress impacts the secretion of certain hormones, including the sex hormones.
- When stress goes far beyond the person's control, the situation becomes terrifying for the parasympathetic mechanism of the nervous system. This leads to involuntary urination (rushing to the washroom) and also stools.

RESEARCH

A survey by the Society of Homeopaths in the UK found that 87 per cent of patients reported positive changes after homeopathic treatment for stress-related issues.

Another study involved a group of people with above-average levels of stressful anxiety. They were assigned to either a placebo group or a group receiving a combination of homeopathic remedies to relieve anxiety. The results showed that homeopathy produced significantly better outcomes than the placebo.

In a clinical study, a group of students experiencing test-induced stress and anxiety received either a homeopathic medicine or a placebo. The students taking the homeopathic medicine experienced a significant reduction in test-induced anxiety compared to those who received the placebo.

These studies suggest that homeopathy offers effective relief for stress-related conditions and anxiety.[4]

HEALING WITH HOMEOPATHY

Stress	Homeopathic Remedy
Precipitating Factors	
Bad news	*Calcarea carbonicum*
Broken love affair	*Ignatia amara*
Business failure	*Ambra grisea*
Business worries	*Nux vomica*
Death of near and dear ones	*Natrum muriaticum*
Examination	*Gelsemium sempervirens*
Financial loss	*Rhus toxicodendron*
Good news	*Coffea cruda*
Homesickness	*Phosphoricum acidum*
In men, from domination	*Lycopodium clavatum*
In women, from domination	*Sepia officinalis*
Insult	*Staphysagria*
Jealousy	*Lachesis muta*
Money matters	*Bryonia alba*
Overwork	*Acid picricum*
Post-delivery	*Pulsatilla nigricans*
Stage fright	*Silicea*
Associated With	
Annoyance, irritability	*Nux vomica*
Anxiety	*Argentum nitricum*
Shock	*Aconite napellus*
Silence	*Natrum muriaticum*
Weeping	*Pulsatilla nigricans*

Dose: 30C pills, twice a day until symptoms subside.
Please consult your doctor before starting medication.
Specific remedy: *Kalium phosphoricum* 6X, 3–4 tablets every two hours, until symptoms subside.

CASE STUDY

Case 1

Simran, a 27-year-old woman, approached us with generalised hair loss. The volume of her hair had reduced considerably over a period of six months. She had no other health concern. On a detailed case analysis, we found that Simran was going through a stressful phase. Her father, to whom she was extremely attached, had recently passed away after prolonged illness. She was very depressed since then, though she would not express her feelings openly. She would often weep in solitude and curb her interactions with others.

We prescribed her the homeopathic remedy *Natrum muriaticum*. In a span of three months, it helped her overcome her grief and brought her life back on track. She began to experience significant reduction in hair loss, and the volume of hair on her scalp gradually returned to normal.

Case 2

Mihir, a 34-year-old man, suffered from excess stress, apprehension and depression and had anxiety spells with profuse sweating of the palms and feet—his sweat would drip like a hydrant. More than stress, Mihir reported that his excessive sweating with damp hands, feet and armpits often created embarrassment. It made him freeze before a handshake and he was uncomfortable at the workplace and during social interactions. This also led to his stressful depressive spells.

Mihir was prescribed *Argentum nitricum* based on his symptoms. After treatment and regular follow-ups for a period of one year, Mihir reported that he was feeling less stressful and anxious and had never felt better any time before. He had comparatively dry, confident hands thanks to homeopathic treatment.

SELF-HELP

- Find out the reason causing distress, write down the cause, thoughts and mood.
- Before you react, reconsider the situation.
- Exercise increases the production of endorphins, your body's natural mood-booster.
- Sleep adequately.
- Limit caffeine intake.
- Restrict screen time.
- Activities like yoga and relaxation exercises not only help reduce stress but also boost immune functioning.
- Focus on something you love doing.
- Put on some music sing and dance along.
- Limit your responsibilities.

Acknowledgements

To write a book on mental health indeed takes a lot of mental effort. This book would not have been possible without the help of a few members of my team. Let me start with my ever-reliable and dependable assistant Louisa for having proofread the book. A special thanks to my colleague Dr Tanvi Lokhande for her research on the topic. This book would not have seen the light of day had it not been for the effort of Mita Kapur and my literary agency SIYAHI for having put me in touch with Bloomsbury. A big thank you to the wonderful team at Bloomsbury—Krishan Chopra, Meenakshi Singh, Mekhala Moorthy and Sanjiv Sarin—who painstakingly worked on this book.

I hope that this book helps you or someone you know who is suffering from mental health issues to lead a healthier and happier life.

Appendix

How to Take, Select, Use and Store Homeopathic Medicines

HOW TO TAKE HOMEOPATHIC MEDICINES

Homeopathic medicines should be kept under the tongue in a clean mouth, preferably about half an hour before or after meals. You should avoid drinking coffee for about half an hour before taking homeopathic medicines (tea, however, is okay). Do not consume homeopathic medicines after using a toothpaste with mint flavour to brush your teeth or after using a medicinal/cosmetic mouthwash.

When taking homeopathic pills or tablets, handle them carefully. Take them directly; don't use the palm of your hands. If any pills fall on the ground, discard them.

The best way to consume homeopathic pills is to dissolve them under the tongue or suck them; don't swallow them whole. Avoid eating or drinking or brushing your teeth (with toothpaste) for 30 minutes before as well as after taking a homeopathic remedy.

Children may find this difficult to follow. But don't give them homeopathic pills with food. For children (especially autistic kids) who don't take pills or spit them out, just crush the pills on a clean, dry spoon and administer the powder. The same procedure can be followed while giving homeopathic pills to your pets or animals.

SELECTING THE REMEDY

You may have taken homeopathic medicines earlier. If you have, you will know the importance your homeopathic physician attaches to your symptoms and case history. The physician would have asked several probing questions. Your responses and your physician's reading of your case would have decided the treatment best suited for you. This may or may not relate to a number of different and/or apparently unrelated conditions—as they may appear to a layperson. Symptoms such as 'being worse at night', or 'better in the open air', or 'after food' or 'before food' can lead the physician to the correct remedy.

The homeopathic remedies presented in this book are chosen keeping the common requirements in mind. They are most useful to treat disorders in the average home situation of readers who have relatively straightforward symptoms. What's more, these remedies are safe and easy to use.

To begin with, you should rely on the description of the symptoms given for each disorder in this book. Just stick to the basics. Keep it simple. Once you do this, you will be able to prescribe the remedies, with fairly good effect. Remember, homeopathic medicines work best when you address the individual as one whole, not just the illness alone. In other words, evaluating the individual's physical, mental and emotional planes simultaneously is required.

Once you get a good feel of it, you will be able to refer to the Materia Medica to connect with the main pattern of symptoms with a suitable remedy.

The blueprint of symptoms in a remedy is called the symptom picture. It holds the key to effective homeopathic prescribing.

A remedy that closely matches its symptom picture with the symptoms of the individual, with a given or not given illness, is known in homeopathy as the *similimum*. In other words, this is the most similar remedy. When the match is correct, the medicinal action is often impressive and satisfying. This is the hallmark of correct prescribing—when you do it, you will know its results. Because seeing is believing.

DOSAGE

Most often, homeopathic medicines are given in pills form, to be placed under the tongue and allowed to dissolve. These are small, round pills, easy to consume. They can be packed in small bottles and can last for long periods. The usual dose is 5–6 pills for an adult and a child alike.

A normal dose of any homeopathic medicine in liquid form is 8–10 drops, dissolved in half a cup of water. The medicinal liquid can be rubbed into the chest when the individual cannot open the mouth. In extremely acute cases, put half a capful, or about 20 drops, in some water in a glass, and take a few teaspoonfuls at a time, at half-hour intervals.

In most acute illnesses, a dose may be taken every 2–3 hours during the day. This may be continued at night if the individual is awake.

Homeopathic medicines in tablet form are also available. They may be placed under the tongue and allowed to dissolve, or they can be chewed, if preferred. The usual dose is 4–6 tablets for adults, 3–4 tablets for children.

Oral sprays are a new introduction in homeopathic practice. They have proved to be convenient in children and older adults. The usual dose is 4–5 sprays for an adult, 2–3 sprays for a child.

Dosages and repetitions depend on the potency used, the type of illness and the age of the patient.

As a general rule of the thumb, low potencies—6X, or 3C to 12C—are used in acute conditions such as colds, headaches, vomiting, injuries and wounds.

Medium potencies such as 30C or 200C are used in more established conditions like recurring migraines or menstrual periods.

Higher potencies—1M and above—are best used in deeper constitutional illnesses and treatment, under the guidance of a trained homeopathic physician.

It may be borne in mind that 6X and 6C are good, fast-acting potencies. They are also best suited for most common health disorders. They are available in a variety of dose forms, including liquids, pills and tablets.

REPETITION

One dose of 3X–6X potency may be given until the patient improves or until a change occurs. If there is no change after one or two weeks, in acute illnesses, it may be deduced that the remedy has failed. It's time to move on to a new remedy.

Most homeopaths repeat medium potencies—30C and 200C—once or twice a day for adults and children for several days. This is done in long-term disorders such as arthritis or constipation for several weeks.

For chronic conditions, the 200 C potency may be given once a week. Higher potencies, such as 1M, are given every month for constitutional illnesses.

It is seen that infants and children respond more quickly to remedies than adults. This happens despite the fact that their symptom picture often changes quickly. It is recommended that they should be monitored closely. This is particularly applicable for infants, where results from a single dose can appear within a few minutes and up to an hour. This suggests that infants may be given doses less often, probably once in the morning and once at bedtime.

Wait. Watch. Act

It is always good to wait for some time after giving a well-chosen remedy to elicit a response. You may encounter the following three situations after giving the medicine and after waiting for results to emerge.

When symptoms improve (ameliorate)

When symptoms disappear and the individual feels better, there is no need to repeat the medicine. You may give a repeat dose only when the improvement stops or when there is no further progress.

When symptoms persist

The remedy has failed when there is no improvement after 6–8 hours, or 3–4 days in acute conditions. You will then have to select a new remedy.

When symptoms worsen (aggravate)

Probably the remedy you've given is well chosen, but it may have overstimulated a response. Just stop the medicine.

Most often, a marked improvement is seen once the homeopathic aggravation subsides. You may have to repeat a dose or two, if there is no progress—not otherwise. If the earlier improvement stops and there is a lull, you may switch over to a higher potency than what you started with.

When the aggravation state does not ebb, it is best to seek professional advice. It may be borne in mind that any illness that fails to improve after the administration of well-chosen remedies should always be reviewed by a trained homeopathic physician in an office consultation.

HOW TO STORE HOMEOPATHIC MEDICINES

Homeopathic medicines can be preserved for long periods of time (up to three years, or more). They don't lose their medicinal strength. However, the bottles/containers should be closed securely and stored in a cool, dark place like a cupboard or a drawer.

Keep the medicines away from direct sunlight, strong odours, perfumes and liniments.

Homeopathic medicines don't need refrigeration.

Keep them away from microwave ovens, electronic gadgets and computers.

Keep medicines away from:

- Coffee powder, tea and drugs having a high caffeine content
- Camphor (mothballs, balms, ointments with cooling or heating effects, lipstick)
- Mint (e.g., in toothpaste), chewing gum
- Ethereal oils (clove oil, eucalyptus, peppermint, menthol)
- Daily or prolonged exposure to strong-smelling substances like paints, glue, varnishes
- Alcohol, spicy food (spices contain ethereal oils)
- Fresh garlic and onion

Notes

Introduction

1 TNN, 'India Is World's Suicide Capital with 2.6 Lakh Cases/ Year', *Times of India*, 5 September 2014, https://timesofindia.indiatimes.com/india/india-is-worlds-suicide-capital-with-2-6-lakh-cases/year/articleshow/41737654.cms.

2 Ruchi Jain, 'World Mental Health Day: 60-70 Mn People in India Suffer from Common Mental Disorders; Stigmatisation & Financial Barriers Prevent Timely Treatment', *Economic Times*, 10 October 2023, https://economictimes.indiatimes.com/magazines/panache/world-mental-health-day-60-70-mn-people-in-india-suffer-from-common-mental-disorders-stigmatisation-financial-barriers-prevent-timely-treatment/articleshow/104289268.cms.

Chapter 1 Anxiety

1 'History of Anxiety Disorders', *eTherapy*, 4 January 2021, https://etherapypro.com/history-of-anxiety-disorders/.

2 'Anxiety', *American Psychological Association*, https://www.apa.org/topics/anxiety.

3 Naziya Nawab, 'Mental Health Care Analysis', *Times of India*, 7 October 2022, https://timesofindia.indiatimes.com/blogs/voices/mental-health-care-analysis/.

4 'Why Many Indians Don't Trust Mental Health Advice', The Wire, 3 June 2023, https://thewire.in/society/why-many-indians-dont-trust-mental-health-advice.

5 'Anxiety Disorders', World Health Organization, 27 September 2023, https://www.who.int/news-room/fact-sheets/detail/anxiety-disorders.

6 'Anxiety Disorders', Cleveland Clinic, https://my.clevelandclinic.org/health/diseases/9536-anxiety-disorders.
7 Jon Cooper, Medically reviewed by Poonam Sachdev, 'Anxiety vs. Insomnia', WebMD, 19 September 2023, https://www.webmd.com/sleep-disorders/anxiety-vs-insomnia.
8 'Treating Addiction with Anxiety Disorders', *American Addiction Centers*, 29 June 2023, https://americanaddictioncenters.org/anxiety-and-addiction.
9 Lamiae Grimaldi-Bensouda, et al., 'Homeopathic Medical Practice for Anxiety and Depression in Primary Care: The EPI3 Cohort Study', *BMC Complementary Medicine and Therapies*, 4 May 2016, https://bmccomplementmedtherapies.biomedcentral.com/articles/10.1186/s12906-016-1104-2.
10 'Exercise for Stress and Anxiety', ADAA, https://adaa.org/living-with-anxiety/managing-anxiety/exercise-stress-and-anxiety.

Chapter 2 Depression

1 'The History of Depression', Brains Way, https://www.brainsway.com/knowledge-center/the-history-of-depression/.
2 Mara Santilli, Medically reviewed by Sabrina Romanoff, 'Depression Statistics in 2023', *Forbes Health*, https://www.forbes.com/health/mind/depression-statistics/.
3 'What Happens to the Brain During Depression?' Transformations Treatment Center, https://www.transformationstreatment.center/treatment/what-happens-to-the-brain- during- depression/.
4 'Depression and Sleep: Understanding the Connection', Johns Hopkins Medicine, https://www.hopkinsmedicine.org/health/wellness-and-prevention/depression-and-sleep-understanding-the-connection.
5 'Depression and Suicide', Cincinnati Children's, https://www.cincinnatichildrens.org/health/d/depression-suicide.
6 David S. Spence, Elizabeth A. Thompson and S.J. Barron, 'Homeopathic Treatment for Chronic Disease: A 6-Year, University-Hospital Outpatient Observational Study, National Library of Medicine, October 2005, https://pubmed.ncbi.nlm.nih.gov/16296912/.

7 'Homeopathy & Depression', Dr Batra's, https://www.drbatras.com/homeopathy-depression.
8 https://www.who.int/news-room/fact-sheets/detail/mental-health-at-work
9 Wyatt Myers, '7 Great Exercises to Ease Depression', Everyday Health, 4 August 2023, https://www.everydayhealth.com/depression-pictures/great-exercises-to-fight-depression.aspx.

Chapter 3 Eating Disorders

1 Antoni Niedzielski, Natalia Kazmierczak and Andrzej Grzybowski, 'Sir William Withey Gull (1816–1890)', National Library of Medicine, 8 August 2016, https://www.ncbi.nlm.nih.gov/pmc/articles/PMC5306080/.
2 'Eating Disorder Awareness Week in India', SKOOC, 13 March 2023, https://www.skooc.com/blog/eating-disorder-awareness-week-in-india-2023.
3 'Neurotransmitters', NEDA, https://www.nationaleatingdisorders.org/toolkit/parent-toolkit/neurotransmitters.
4 'Eating Disorder Awareness Week in India', SKOOC, 13 March 2023, https://www.skooc.com/blog/eating-disorder-awareness-week-in-india-2023.
5 'Bulimia Nervosa', United Brain Association, https://unitedbrainassociation.org/brain-resources/bulimia-nervosa/.
6 'Bulimia Nervosa', United Brain Association, https://unitedbrainassociation.org/brain-resources/bulimia-nervosa/.
7 'What We Treat', Walden, https://www.waldeneatingdisorders.com/what-we-treat/bulimia/.
8 'What We Treat', Walden, https://www.waldeneatingdisorders.com/what-we-treat/bulimia/.
9 Hertzog Johannes van Heerden, Radmila Razlog and Janice Pellow, 'Pilot Study on the Homeopathic Treatment of Binge Eating in Males', PubMed, April 2016, https://pubmed.ncbi.nlm.nih.gov/27089525/.
10 'Malnutrition', World Health Organization, 9 June 2021, https://www.who.int/news-room/fact-sheets/detail/malnutrition.
11 'Dieting', Wikipedia, https://en.wikipedia.org/wiki/Dieting.
12 'World Obesity Day 2023: Is India Battling an Obesity Epidemic?' News 18, 4 March 2023, https://www.news18.com/

news/lifestyle/world-obesity-day-2023-is-india-battling-an-obesity-epidemic-7216951.html.

13 'Obesity', World Heart Federation, https://world-heart-federation.org/what-we-do/obesity/.

14 'Obesity', World Heart Federation, https://world-heart-federation.org/what-we-do/obesity/.

15 Geeta Pandey, 'NFHS-5: Indians Are Getting Fatter—and It's a Big Problem', BBC News, 25 May 2022, https://www.bbc.com/news/world-asia-india-61558119.

16 Chemin Eugene, 'A Different Scale: Global Action to Address Obesity', World Health Organization, 24 May 2022, https://www.who.int/news-room/events/detail/2022/05/24/default-calendar/a-different-scale-global-action-to-address-obesity.

17 S. Sharma and Pranesh Kumar Singh, 'Management of Obesity with Homoeopathy—A Review', ResearchGate, October 2019, https://www.researchgate.net/publication/336578148.

Chapter 4 Attention Deficit Hyperactivity Disorder (ADHD)

1 Prosenjit Ghosh, Hasina Anjuman Choudhury and Robin Victor, 'Prevalence of Attention Deficit Hyperactivity Disorder among Primary School Children in Cachar, Assam, North-East India', ResearchGate, July 2018, https://www.researchgate.net/publication/326474503.

2 https://linkprotect.cudasvc.com/url?a=https%3a%2f%2fwww.indiatoday.in%2fscience%2fstory%2findian-herb-saffron-can-replace-stimulant-medicine-for-treating-adhd-in-children-1463600-2019-02-24&c=E,1,2bXPQ4vAPy6oHDr5B5MBG8641A2fFMrd1EY1ASrvRf1aa3hNtF4ENknsGLloJspiR43WCFZjuWy3N1kUufqdmjFiK3Uv6JoJFV7PG9_yeINAKaGvimmxblY ,&typo= 1

2 Heiner Frei, Regula Everts, Klaus von Ammon and Franz Kaufmann, 'Homeopathic Treatment of Children with Attention Deficit Hyperactivity Disorder: A Randomised, Double Blind, Placebo Controlled Crossover Trial', ResearchGate, December 2005, https://www.researchgate.net/publication/7698856.

Chapter 5 Obsessions

1 'National Mental Health Survey of India, 2015-16', National Institute of Mental Health and Neurosciences, Bengaluru, 2016, https://main.mohfw.gov.in/sites/default/files/National%20Mental%20Health%20Survey%2C%202015-16%20-%20Mental%20Health%20Systems_0.pdf.
2 Karunakara Moorthi, Susu Pertin and Radhika Prasannakumar, 'Homoeopathy for Obsessive-Compulsive Disorder: A Case Report', ResearchGate, June 2023, https://www.researchgate.net/publication/371947557.

Chapter 6 Fears

1 Helen Chao, 'Phobia through the Ages', *El Estoque*, 13 September 2017, https://elestoque.org/2017/09/13/special/verge-phobia-ages/.
2 J.K. Trivedi and Pawan Kumar Gupta, 'An Overview of Indian Research in Anxiety Disorders', *Indian Journal of Psychiatry*, January 2010, https://www.ncbi.nlm.nih.gov/pmc/articles/PMC3146193/.
3 Heidi Moawad, 'Phobias and Brain Activity', *Neurology Live*, 26 October 2017, https://www.neurologylive.com/view/phobias-and-brain-activity.
4 Deepthi Gilla, et al., 'A Review on Anxiety Disorders During Covid-19 Pandemic: Homoeopathic Perspective', *International Journal of High Dilution Research*, 2021, https://pdfs.semanticscholar.org/0510/cb217736fc14b1f4830f80138dc3b03392cf.pdf.

Chapter 7 Anger

1 'Anger's Alterations', *The Etymology Nerd*, https://www.etymologynerd.com/blog/angers-alterations.
2 'Anger Management', *Wikipedia*, https://en.wikipedia.org/wiki/Anger_management#.
3 Tanvir Kaur Sidhu, et al., 'Aggression among Adolescents: A Cross-Sectional Study', ResearchGate, December 2019, https://www.researchgate.net/publication/338240988.
4 Jack Kelly, 'Global Emotions Survey Shows Record High Levels of People "Feeling Stressed, Sad, Angry and Worried"', Forbes, 31 July 2021, https://www.forbes.com/sites/jackkelly/2021/07/31/

global-emotions-survey-shows-record-high-levels-of-people-feeling-stressed-sad-angry-and-worried/.

5 Christopher Ingraham, *Washington Post*, 8 April 2015, 'Nearly 1 in 10 Americans Have Severe Anger Issues and Access to Guns', Mass. General Hospital, https://clbb.mgh.harvard.edu/nearly-1-in-10-americans-have-severe-anger-issues-and-access-to-guns/.

6 Debbie Strong, '7 Ways Anger Is Ruining Your Health', Everyday Health, 29 May 2015, https://www.everydayhealth.com/news/ways-anger-ruining-your-health/.

7 Lewis L. Judd, et al., 'Overt Irritability/Anger in Unipolar Major Depressive Episodes', JAMA Psychiatry, 2013, https://jamanetwork.com/journals/jamapsychiatry/fullarticle/1737169.

8 'Lack of Sleep Intensifies Anger, Impairs Adaptation to Frustrating Circumstances', Iowa State University News Service, 27 November 2018, https://www.news.iastate.edu/news/2018/11/27/sleepanger.

9 Ambita Maletha and Manoj Kumar Behera, 'Sweet Pills Can Help in Anger Management', ResearchGate, September 2020, https://www.researchgate.net/publication/344382542.

10 Dongju Seo, Christopher J. Patrick and Patrick J. Kennealy, 'Role of Serotonin and Dopamine System Interactions in the Neurobiology of Impulsive Aggression and Its Comorbidity with Other Clinical Disorders, National Library of Medicine, October 2008, https://www.ncbi.nlm.nih.gov/pmc/articles/PMC2612120/.

Chapter 8 Emotional Disorders in Children, Teens and Seniors

1 Rekha Mittal, 'Letters to the Editor: Management of Breath Holding Spells', Indian Pediatrics, 1999, https://www.indianpediatrics.net/mar1999/mar-325-326.htm.

2 'Breath-Holding Spells', Wikipedia, https://en.wikipedia.org/wiki/Breath-holding_spell.

3 Deborah Kotz, 'Nearly 1 in 12 Teens Has Anger Disorder, Harvard Study Finds', Boston, 3 July 2012, https://www.boston.com/uncategorized/noprimarytagmatch/2012/07/03/nearly-1-in-12-teens-has-anger-disorder-harvard-study-finds/.

4 'History of Attachment Theory', Wikipedia, https://en.wikipedia.org/wiki/History_of_attachment_theory.

5 'Reactive Attachment Disorder', Cleveland Clinic, https://my.clevelandclinic.org/health/diseases/17904-reactive-attachment-disorder.
6 Julietta A. Sheng, et al., 'The Hypothalamic–Pituitary–Adrenal Axis: Development, Programming Actions of Hormones, and Maternal–Fetal Interactions', *Frontiers*, 13 January 2021, https://www.frontiersin.org/articles/10.3389/fnbeh.2020.601939/full.
7 Ilana Rosenberg, 'Mother Baby Attachment', 6 November 2013, https://ilanarosenberg.com/2013/11/06/mother-baby-attachment/#:~:text=Bowlby%20developed%20attachment%20theory%20from,instinctual%20drives%20by%20the%20mother.
8 'A Short Cultural History of Bedwetting Treatment', Therapee, https://www.bedwettingtherapy.com/blog/a-short-cultural-history-of-bedwetting-treatment/.
9 N.M. Reddy, et al., 'Nocturnal Enuresis in India: Are We Diagnosing and Managing Correctly?', ResearchGate, May 2017, https://www.researchgate.net/publication/317063575.
10 Matthew Hoffman, Medically reviewed by Roy Benaroch, 'Bedwetting: What Causes It?', WebMD, 25 February 2012, https://www.webmd.com/children/features/bedwetting-causes.
11 Sangita Saha, Rumsha Tamkeen and Subhranil Saha, 'An Open Observational Trial Evaluating the Role of Individualised Homoeopathic Medicines in the Management of Nocturnal Enuresis', ResearchGate, January 2018, https://www.researchgate.net/publication/327888062.
12 Miriam Brazzelli, et al. (eds), 'Behavioural and Cognitive Interventions with or without Other Treatments for the Management of Faecal Incontinence in Children', National Library of Medicine, 7 December 2011, https://www.ncbi.nlm.nih.gov/pmc/articles/PMC7103956/.
13 Luis Villazon, 'What's the Longest Time that Somebody Has Been Constipated?', BBC Science Focus, https://www.sciencefocus.com/the-human-body/whats-the-longest-time-that-somebody-has-been-constipated.
14 Mohanty Nimain and Rishabh Dutt, 'Diagnosis and Management of Chronic Constipation', *New Indian*

Journal of Pediatrics, April–June 2015, https://nijp.org/diagnosis-and-management-of-chronic-constipation/.

15 Suzannah Showler, 'Letter of Recommendation: Nail-Biting', *New York Times Magazine*, 23 October 2018, https://www.nytimes.com/2018/10/23/magazine/letter-of-recommendation-nail-biting.html.

16 'Nail Biting Can Really Give You a Disease', *Times of India*, 6 June 2015, https://timesofindia.indiatimes.com/life-style/health-fitness/health-news/nail-biting-can-really-give-you-a-disease/articleshow/17227999.cms.

17 'How to Manage Adult Thumb-Sucking', Zombek Orthodontics, https://www.zombekortho.com/adult-thumb-sucking/.

18 Lynn Davidson, 'Thumb and Finger Sucking', American Academy of Pediatrics, 1 June 2018, https://publications.aap.org/pediatricsinreview/article-abstract/29/6/207/33967/.

19 Genie Rowson, 'Homeopathy for Behaviour Disorders in Kids', news24, 21 May 2012, https://www.news24.com/life/archive/homeopathy-for-behaviour-disorders-in-kids-20120721.

20 Linda Rodriguez McRobbie, 'The History of Boredom', *Smithsonian Magazine*, 20 November 2012, https://www.smithsonianmag.com/science-nature/the-history-of-boredom-138176427/.

21 Meghan E. Martz, et al., '"I Am So Bored!": Prevalence Rates and Sociodemographic and Contextual Correlates of High Boredom among American Adolescents', *Sage Journals*, 9 February 2016, https://journals.sagepub.com/doi/abs/10.1177/0044118X15626624?journalCode=yasa.

22 PTI, 'Indians Snack More amid Pandemic to Overcome Boredom', *Business Today*, 11 December 2020, https://www.businesstoday.in/latest/trends/story/indians-snack-more-amid-pandemic-to-overcome-boredom-281283-2020-12-11.

23 Carla Cantor, 'Why Being Bored Can Be Hazardous to Your Health', *Columbia News*, 8 November 2019, https://news.columbia.edu/news/why-being-bored-can-be-hazardous-your-health.

24 Ibid.

25 Maria Cohut, 'What Happens in the Brain When We Are Bored?' *MedicalNewsToday*, 9 July 2019, https://www.medicalnewstoday.com/articles/325697#The-study-premises

26 'Olwes Bullying Prevention Program', Olwes, https://olweus.sites.clemson.edu/history.php.
27 Priyanka Sangani, '85% of Indian Children Have Been Cyberbullied, Highest Globally: McAfee', *Economic Times*, 9 August 2022, https://economictimes.indiatimes.com/tech/technology/85-of-indian-children-have-been-cyberbullied-highest-globally-mcafee/articleshow/93438743.cms?from=mdr.
28 Ignatius Pereira, 'India Saw 1,35,445 Suicides Last Year', *The Hindu*, 25 June 2013, https://www.thehindu.com/news/national/india-saw-135445-suicides-last-year/article4849710.ece.
29 'Divorce Statistics for 2022', Petrelli Previtera, 1 September 2023, https://www.petrellilaw.com/divorce-statistics-for-2022/.
30 'The History of Depression', BrainsWay, https://www.brainsway.com/knowledge-center/the-history-of-depression/.
31 Nancy Schimelpfening, 'The History of Depression', verywell mind, https://www.verywellmind.com/who-discovered-depression-1066770.
32 Manju Pilania, et al., 'Prevalence of Depression among the Elderly (60 Years and Above) Population in India, 1997–2016: A Systematic Review and Meta-Analysis', BMC Public Health, 19, 832 (2019), https://doi.org/10.1186/s12889-019-7136-z.
33 'Health Issues', HHCC, https://hhcc.com.au/health-issues/.
34 'Milestones', Alzheimer's Association, https://www.alz.org/alzheimers-dementia/research_progress/milestones.
35 Jui Dharwadkar, 'India Has Second Most Number of Individuals Suffering from Dementia', *Hindustan Times*, 20 September 2017, https://www.hindustantimes.com/pune-news/india-has-second-most-number-of-individuals-suffering-from-dementia/story-FpMAyRUxeq2yVuVngHtpSM.html.
36 Kashif Hanif, et al., 'Effect of Homeopathic Lycopodium Clavatum on Memory Functions and Cerebral Blood Flow in Memory-Impaired Rats', ResearchGate, October 2014, https://www.researchgate.net/publication/267159419.

Chapter 9 Lack of Confidence

1 Mohnish Nelarwar, '90% People Have Low Self-Esteem: Experts', *Times of India*, 12 September 2017, https://timesofindia.

indiatimes.com/city/nagpur/90-people-have-low-self-esteem-experts/articleshow/60469457.cms.

Chapter 10 Loneliness

1 David Riesman, Nathan Glazer and Reuel Denney, *The Lonely Crowd: A Study of the Changing American Character*, 1 March 2001, https://www.amazon.com/Lonely-Crowd-Revised-Changing-Character/dp/0300088655?ots=1&tag=thneyooof-20&linkCode=w50.

2 Aparna Shankar and Tara Kidd, 'Loneliness in Older Indian Dyads', National Library of Medicine, 27 April 2022, https://www.ncbi.nlm.nih.gov/pmc/articles/PMC9101006/.

3 American Heart Association Scientific Statement, 'Social Isolation and Loneliness Increase the Risk of Death from Heart Attack, Stroke', Newsroom, 4 August 2022, https://newsroom.heart.org/news/social-isolation-and-loneliness-increase-the-risk-of-death-from-heart-attack-stroke.

4 'UN Leads Call to Protect Most Vulnerable from Mental Health Crisis During and after COVID-19', UN News, 14 May 2020, https://news.un.org/en/story/2020/05/1063882.

Chapter 11 Loneliness

1 Banavaram Anniappan Arvind, et al., 'Prevalence and Socioeconomic Impact of Depressive Disorders in India: Multisite Population-Based Cross-Sectional Study', National Library of Medicine, 27 June 2019, https://www.ncbi.nlm.nih.gov/pmc/articles/PMC6609075/.

2 'What Is Mood Swings?' Medicover Hospitals, 26 February 2021, https://www.medicoverhospitals.in/symptoms/mood-swings.

3 Colette Bouchez, Medically reviewed by Brunilda Nazario, 'Serotonin: 9 Questions and Answers', WebMD, 12 October 2011, https://www.webmd.com/depression/features/serotonin.

4 Audrey J. Brooks, et al., 'Effects of Homeopathic Medicines on Mood of Adults with Histories of Coffee-Related Insomnia', National Library of Medicine, 1 October 2010, https://pubmed.ncbi.nlm.nih.gov/20980764/.

Chapter 12 Stress and How to Manage It

1 'What Is Stress?' American Institute of Stress, https://www.stress.org/what-is-stress.
2 '24% of Indians Are Struggling with Stress: Report', *Deccan Herald*, 6 March 2023, https://www.deccanherald.com/business/24-of-indians-are-struggling-with-stress-report-1197723.html.
3 'The Science behind Stress and How to Relieve the Symptoms', Burkhart Dental, https://www.burkhartdental.com/wp-content/uploads/2020/04/The-Science-Behind-Stress-and-How-to-Relieve-the-Symptoms.pdf.
4 'Homeopathy & Stress', Dr Batras, https://www.drbatras.com/homeopathy-stress.

About the Author

Dr Mukesh Batra is the founder and chairman of Dr Batra's® Healthcare—the world's largest chain of homeopathy clinics with over 225 clinics across six countries. His foundation helps the underprivileged with free homeopathy treatment at over 175 clinics and offers scholarships to students at ten of India's leading homeopathy colleges.

He has been granted honorary fellowships by homeopathy colleges in the US and the UK. He is also a patron of the Trichological Society, UK, one of the world's oldest hair specialist institutions. Dr Batra is a member of the national task force and the co-chair for AYUSH, Homeopathy, of the Confederation of Indian Industry. He is also a member of the advisory board of the Chamber of Fair Business Practices. He is the president of SKAL Mumbai, South, an industry body of hospitality.

Dr Batra was awarded the Padma Shri, one of India's highest civilian awards, in 2012 for Medicine, Homeopathy, by the President of India. He has authored ten bestselling books on homeopathy with international publishing houses.